The Food and Mood Handbook

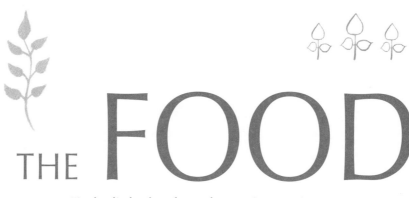

THE FOOD AND MOOD

Find relief at last from depression, anxiety, PMS, cravings and mood swings

HANDBOOK

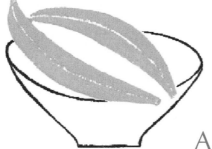

AMANDA GEARY

Thorsons

Thorsons
An Imprint of HarperCollins*Publishers*
77–85 Fulham Palace Road
Hammersmith, London W6 8JB

The Thorsons website address is www.thorsons.com

Published by Thorsons 2001

10 9 8 7 6 5 4

© Amanda Geary 2001

Amanda Geary asserts the moral right to
be identified as the author of this work

Cartoons reproduced by kind permission of Angela Martin
Illustrations by Peter Cox Associates, Jennie Dooge and Julian Howell

A catalogue record for this book is
available from the British Library

ISBN 0 00 711423 0

Printed and bound in Great Britain by
Scotprint, Haddington

For Padraig. Also for my parents, Keith and Sheila, and my sisters, Joanne and Rachel.

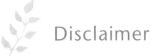

Disclaimer

This handbook is intended as a source of information only and not as an alternative to medical advice. While every care is taken in preparing this material, the author or publishers cannot accept any responsibility for any damage or harm caused by any treatment, advice or information contained in this publication. You should consult a qualified medical practitioner before undertaking any treatment. Unless a statement is specifically referenced, it could be the author's opinion, based on extensive study and personal experience. The Further Reading section in Resources contains many of the sources used to research this book.

Acknowledgements

I would like to thank Mind and the Millennium Commission for the Mind Millennium Award grant that made the original Food and Mood Project possible. Les Moore and Fiona Saunders at Natural Health Foods/Wholefood Express in Brighton for providing the original home for the Project.

The members of the British Association of Nutritional Therapists (BANT) who kindly contributed case material, including June Butlin, Julie Green, Heather Lyons, Pat Reeves, Veronica Wolesley. Julian Howell for his brilliant design work on the original Workbook (some of which has been used for this Handbook) and his continuing work for the Food and Mood Project. Angela Martin for her wonderfully appropriate cartoons, and the inspiration gained from the excellent resource pack 'Women, Food & Health' published by Mancunian Community Nutrition. Johnny Denis and Sarah Davies of C.A.F.E. at East Sussex, Brighton & Hove Health Promotion for the inspiration behind the 'recipe for change' used in Chapter 10. A special thank you to Padraig Breatnach for his careful scrutiny of the manuscript and insightful comments. Thanks also to Rachel Geary for her comments on the first and final chapters. Also to Bron Grillo and Karen Sargent for their help with the distribution of The Food & Mood Workbook. Thank you to the staff at Equilibrium in Lewes, Sussex and particularly Victoria Cooper who helped to keep me relaxed and de-stressed whilst working on the manuscript.

Most importantly, the 50 or so women who took part in the original Project and the many men and women who continue to attend Food and Mood workshops or for private consultations who are personally investigating the links between diet, nutrition and emotional and mental health.

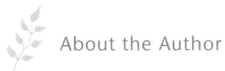

About the Author

Amanda Geary, registered nutritional therapist and founder of the Food and Mood Project, received a Millennium Award from Mind, the UK's leading mental health charity, for the highly successful Food and Mood Project. Amanda, also an experienced complementary therapist, continues to work closely with Mind. She recently created the Mind Meal which was launched in Mind Week 2000 and is author of *The Mind Guide to Food and Mood*, published by Mind.

In addition to her work with the Project, Amanda provides nutritional therapy consultations at private clinics in Brighton and Lewes, Sussex. She also consults for The Children's Clinic at Dolphin House, the innovative UK children's charity for complementary therapies which is pioneering a nutritional therapy outreach service in government-recognized areas of urban deprivation.

Amanda gained the Diploma in Nutritional Counselling from the Raworth Centre, International College for Sports Therapy and Natural Medicine, Dorking, Surrey, and is registered with the British Association of Nutritional Therapists (BANT).

Also by the Author

The Food & Mood Workbook
The Mind Guide to Food and Mood

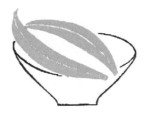

Contents

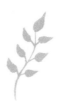

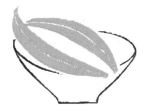

1
Food and Mood

Welcome to The Food and Mood Handbook

This handbook invites you to consider the idea that what you eat can change how you feel. Within its pages you will be able to discover that food is much more than just fuel to keep you going. Food can affect mood, and what you choose to put in your mouth can influence the state of your mind.

This handbook offers tried and tested methods for uncovering the hidden relationship between food and mood. Greater control of your moods and energy levels is possible through exploring the links between diet, nutrition and emotional and mental health. You will be guided to experience first hand the mood-altering effects of food. In this way you will find out what you need to eat to feel good for longer. You may learn that you are not quite the person you thought you were, as symptoms of depression, irritability or anxiety change along with your diet.

The Food and Mood Handbook therefore offers a complementary approach to the treatment of emotional and mental health problems. Whether used in addition, or as an alternative, to drug-based treatments and counselling therapies, food can also be found to be powerful and effective medicine.

Give a person a fish and you feed them for one day; teach someone how to fish and you feed them for a lifetime

This well-known proverb describes the approach of *The Food and Mood Handbook*. For although this handbook contains many ideas and suggestions for how food can improve mood, they are recommendations rather than a prescription. Instead, this handbook provides an opportunity for *you* to become the expert at deciding what is best for *your* mind and body.

How to Use This Handbook

This handbook offers a varied 'menu' of ideas and practical suggestions for you to try. Have a look at what is available and start with whatever appeals the most. If you can share the experience with a friend, so much the better. Feel free to dip in – perhaps use your intuition to guide you. To avoid indigestion, consume the contents slowly and chew well. Then, when you are almost full, stop for a while. Allow yourself time to digest and assimilate what you've absorbed. There is much 'food for thought' for you to try and the remainder will keep well for later on. Bon appetit!

 Relating with the Environment

To stay healthy, our bodies are constantly changing as they work to keep things in balance. The name of this life-sustaining process is homeostasis and it involves an intricate network of bodily checks and balances. Yet our bodies don't work in isolation, for they are also involved in an ongoing relationship with our surroundings, the air we breathe, the water we drink and the food we eat.

Air, food and water are life-giving substances that enter our bodies and become transformed into who we are. The environment also receives and contains the products of that transformation: the air we exhale, the wastes we excrete and the sounds and movements, thoughts and actions of our bodies.

We are not yet fully aware of how intimate is our connection with the environment.

Achieving harmony between what's 'out there' and what's 'inside' is a constant and delicate balancing act. How we feel about this relationship may be reflected in the way we breathe, eat, digest and absorb our foods. By drawing your attention to the link between food and mood, this handbook is suggesting we are not yet fully aware of how intimate is our connection with the environment.

Food as Medicine

'Let food be your medicine and your medicine be your food' said Hippocrates, the 'father of modern medicine', over two thousand years ago. Food is comprised of many natural chemicals. In addition, there are the many artificial chemicals that, nowadays, are often added during food preparation and processing – not all of which may be beneficial to health. Food can even be thought of as a powerful 'medicine' which we are taking, usually several times each day. And like any 'medicine', it is important that we choose a type that will support our physical and mental health rather than undermine it.

My Story

This handbook has been written from my experiences – both personal and professional – and my explorations into the link between diet, nutrition and emotional and mental health. In 1992 I was diagnosed by my doctor as suffering with depression and pre-scribed antidepressant medication together with a programme of cognitive behavioural counselling therapy. I found that the weekly counselling sessions helped my state of mind and I continued with the therapy for some eight months. The antidepressant med-ication I wasn't so sure of and, having taken the medication for one month without noticing any benefits (merely side-effects), I decided to stop taking it.

At the end of the first year of my illness, many symptoms I was experiencing had still not improved. It was at this point that my doctor decided another opinion was needed and I was referred to a consultant neurologist who diagnosed the illness known as ME or CFS (Chronic Fatigue Syndrome). It was an enormous relief for me that my symptoms of fatigue and weakness were being seen as real and not 'all in my mind' but it was to be a few more years before I would make any clear progress.

I had completed my training as a nutritional therapist before becoming ill so I had a lot of useful information inside my head and was enthusiastic about the importance of diet and nutrition. But changing your diet when you are well can be challenging – when you are ill it can be virtually impossible without a lot of help. Therefore, in the months and years following my ME/CFS diagnosis, I was able to make only a few minor adjust-ments to my diet. It was to be some time before I could initiate the larger dietary changes that would prove to be the turning point in my recovery.

These experiences have stayed with me and probably are the reason why I am able to empathize with the people who now come to me for help. They are keen to learn if nutritional therapy can help, but are understandably concerned about the changes that could be demanded of them. This is why I believe it is so important that nutritional therapy clients feel they – and not their therapist – are in control of the healing process. It is why I recommend making changes at a pace that a person is able to sustain alongside the many competing demands of modern life.

These days, some years after I first became ill, my health is much improved. One difference between how I am now and how I was several years ago is that I am much more aware of how food can affect me. I have changed what I eat on a regular basis and any symptoms I do experience can often be linked to something I have chosen to eat. Consequently, I feel more in control of my physical, *and* emotional and mental, health.

What we eat and drink has an important part to play in how we feel – mentally and emotionally as well as physically.

I now have no doubt that what we eat and drink has an important part to play in how we feel – mentally and emotionally as well as physically. This *Food and Mood Handbook* is therefore part of my continuing desire to spread the food and mood message.

Mind and the Food and Mood Project

My knowledge and experience of helping others discover the links between food and mood received a huge boost in 1998 when I won a Millennium Award from Mind, the mental health charity. The Award enabled me to teach courses for women to explore the relationship between what they eat and how they feel. The original Mind-funded project continued for 18 months, providing a total of six 12-week courses which enabled over 50 women to meet and share their food and mood experiences.

Many of the 50 or so women, of different ages and backgrounds, who took part in the project, found that changing what they ate produced positive benefits to their health. These improvements varied from woman to woman but included:

- lower anxiety levels
- less depression
- improvements in mood swings
- fewer cravings
- reductions in the symptoms of PMS (premenstrual syndrome)
- less fatigue.

Some of the information in this handbook comes directly from these Food and Mood Project participants.

Help is at Hand

People are used to consulting nutritional therapists for help with a wide range of physical health problems. As awareness of the food–mood connection grows, nutritional therapists are being asked to help with more emotional and mental health concerns. Although a lot can be achieved working alone, nutritional therapy undertaken with the support of a professional can be very beneficial. The Resources section of this handbook contains details of some nutritional therapy practitioners with particular experience of helping people with emotional difficulties and diagnosed mental health problems.

Food and Mood Case Studies

The Food and Mood Handbook contains several 'real life' case studies. Covering a range of emotional or mental health concerns, each tells the story of someone who has been successful in changing what they eat to improve the way they feel. These case studies have been contributed by practising nutritional therapists (with the permission of their clients) or have come directly from the men and women who have been helped. Names and personal details have been changed to preserve privacy.

Food and Mood

The relationship between food and mood works both ways. How we feel affecting what we choose to eat or drink – mood to food – is generally accepted. What is new for many people is just how easily what we eat can affect our mental functioning – food to mood. Any exploration into diet, nutrition and emotional and mental health needs to take into account both sides of this two-way relationship. The psychological aspects behind what we are choosing to eat need to be considered as well as the effects of food on mood. This handbook contains some thought-provoking and useful exercises for you to try, some of which aim to increase awareness of the emotions associated with eating and drinking. Exercise One is an opportunity for you to think about what food means to you.

Exercise One: Food and You

Find a large piece of plain paper and some coloured pens. Now, without thinking about it too much, draw or write any pictures, symbols or words that come into your mind when you think about food. These may be positive or negative feelings or associations about your relationship with food. Try not to censor what you draw or write – just express whatever comes to mind.

When you find you have finished, reflect on what you have produced. Does your 'picture' convey a generally happy friendship with food, or are there aspects that are not so positive? What would you like to change about your relationship with food? What do you think you need to make the changes happen?

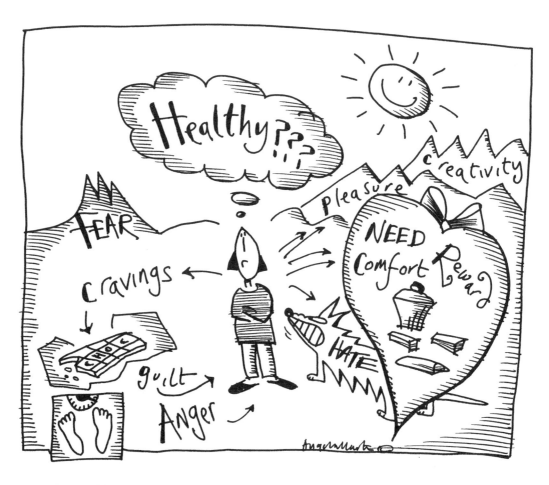

Fig 1 – Food and You

The Mind Food and Mood Survey

A recent survey by the mental health charity Mind reported that nearly nine out of ten people with a range of mental health problems believe there is a link between physical and mental health. Food was found to be an important part of this relationship. A list was compiled of the foods that were thought to have either a positive or negative effect on mood. Foods that were listed (as being either beneficial or detrimental to mental health) included chocolate, sweet or sugary foods, coffee and tea, bread and pasta, fish, chicken, cheese, vegetables and fruit.

The good mood that some people experience from eating sweet or sugary food can soon turn into a bad mood.

An interesting point about this survey which gives the most popular 'good' and 'bad' mood foods is that some foods appear on both lists! For example, at the top of the 'good mood' list was 'sweet or sugary food' because many people find foods like chocolate, biscuits, cake and sweets apparently helpful for improving their moods. However, almost as many people in the survey said that 'sweet or sugary food' had a negative influence on their mental health. The reason these foods appear at the top of both lists is probably because although sugar and chocolate can improve mood for some people, the benefits from these foods are usually felt only in the short term. In other words, the good mood that some people experience from eating sweet or sugary food can soon turn into a bad mood.

Everyone is Unique

Nutritional therapists use the term 'biochemical individuality' to explain the variation between individuals' needs for food and nutrients and it is wise to bear this in mind as you begin to change your diet or take nutritional supplements. The foods that suit your unique biochemistry are unlikely to be exactly the same as the foods that suit your neighbour. 'One person's meat' really can be 'another person's poison'.

Although we can benefit from scientific research and the experiences of other people about what is better (or worse) for us to eat, when exploring the food–mood connection we also need to learn to trust our own judgement. As individuals we each have the power of choice (which we exercise several times each day) over what to eat and drink. As a unique individual only you can directly experience the effect (or not) of a food or drink on your mood. This means that, ultimately, only you can know what is right for you.

Why Change?

Changing what you eat invariably involves eating or drinking less of some things and more of others. But cutting down – and, especially, cutting out – foods can be difficult.

As long as you derive inner help and comfort from anything, you should keep it. If you were to give it up in a mood of self-sacrifice or out of a stern sense of duty, you would continue to want it back, and that unsatisfied want would make trouble for you. Only give up a thing when you want some other condition so much that the thing no longer has any attraction for you.
                                                                                    Gandhi

In other words, it is a lot easier to make changes to what you eat and drink if you hope to benefit in some way from your efforts. And it will be helpful if you can recognize the longer-term benefits as being more important to you than any initial short-term pleasure you might gain from the food you are choosing to give up or cut down on. This hand-book will help you to make informed judgements about the effects of foods, so that you can weigh up the 'costs' and the benefits of making any changes to what you eat and drink.

At this point it may be useful to reflect upon some of your food-and-mood relation-ships, in Exercise Two.

Exercise Two: Food and Mood

Take some time to think about what you eat and drink and if there is an obvious link between the food and the (good or bad) mood that follows. Consider also the (good and bad) moods that influence your choices. This relationship can be quite complex and you may like to summarize your thoughts as a flow chart, something like the one below which takes caffeine as an example:

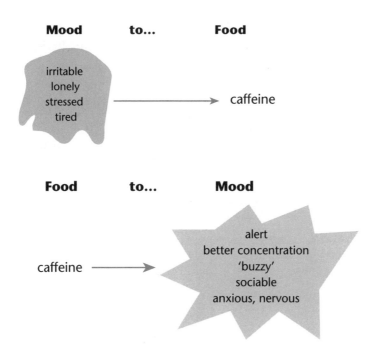

Fig 2 – Food and Mood

Caffeine is found in tea, coffee, cola drinks and chocolate. We often choose to drink it if we are feeling tired and irritable because it seems to give us a boost and helps us to concentrate. Having a cup of coffee or tea also has a lot of positive psychological associations. We meet a friend for a 'coffee and a chat' or give ourselves a break by sitting down with a 'nice cup of tea'. These emotional needs are very important but could be satisfied in other ways, for the consumption of caffeine can have a down side. Too much caffeine, for example, (and this is a different amount for each of us), can cause symptoms such as anxiety, nervousness and depression. *(For more information on caffeine, see Chapter 7).*

The Stressors of Life

Our ability to cope with stress determines how healthy we are. Put another way, our health can be seen as a measure of how well we adapt to the various stressors which are all around us. Stressors are, quite literally, things that can put a stress on a person. If we exceed our capacity to cope with them we begin to fall ill.

It can often help to take a more holistic view and consider the whole picture, as well as looking at individual pieces of the jigsaw.

We each have an intimate relationship with our environment. The association with our surroundings needs to be harmonious if we are to remain healthy. Whilst we search for a solution to the problems of ill health, it can often help to take a more holistic view and consider the whole picture, as well as looking at individual pieces of the jigsaw. The whole picture, when considering our ability to cope with stress and the things that cause us stress, is known as the 'total load'.

The genes we inherited from our parents and the personal characteristics which evolve over time determine our strengths and weaknesses and our ability to cope with, or adapt to, the stressors of life. We can think of our ability to adapt to these stressors as being like a bath, with each of us represented by a different-sized bath.

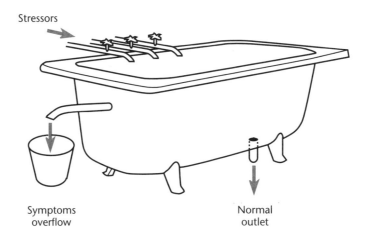

Fig 3 – Bath

Into the bath is flowing all the various influences upon our mental, emotional and physical health. The normal outlet of the bath is unplugged and the bath has the capacity to cope with a certain amount of water without any difficulty. But if the total flow going into the bath – the total load – is more than the bath can contain, then the bath will start to overflow and you will begin to experience symptoms. The greater the overflow from the bath, the worse are the symptoms.

The limit that the bath water has to reach before the bath starts to overflow can be thought of as your personal 'threshold'. Your threshold may change over the course of your life and it is bound to be different to your neighbour's. One person can thrive in a situation that another person finds stressful. What is important to know is your individual capacity for coping, as well as your own personal limits.

As you become more skilled at reading the signs from your body you will find you are able to use quite subtle energy changes to provide information about what is good for you at that particular time.

Symptoms of disease, be they physical, emotional or mental, are a sign that you have exceeded your ability to deal with the total load of stressors in your environment. One of the first signs is loss of energy or a feeling of fatigue. As you become more skilled at reading the signs from your body you will find you are able to use quite subtle energy changes to provide information about what is good for you at that particular time.

A person whose ability to adapt is represented by a deep bath will be someone who is able to cope with a considerable amount of stress before their 'bath' overflows. It will take a lot of water pouring into their bath before they exceed their threshold. When this is reached the bath will start to overflow and this person will experience the early-warning signs and symptoms of ill health. Someone else, who can only manage a relatively low level of stress in their life before feeling overwhelmed, can be thought of as being like a shallow bath. If they are exposed to the same level of stress as the person above, it won't be long before their bath is overflowing and early-warning symptoms of ill health are experienced.

Approaches to health that concentrate on treating symptoms can be thought of as a method of stopping the water from spilling onto the floor – such as putting a bucket under the overflow pipe. Medication that works in this way is represented by the bucket that contains the water. A large bucket represents a large dose of medication. Having to change the bucket at regular intervals is like having to take pills several times a day. The 'bucket approach' to the problem of the overflowing bath does a good job at preventing the water from soaking the carpet and floorboards. But it is clear that, although this method may effectively contain the problem, you have to continue to take the medication (change the bucket). This approach is clearly not addressing the cause of the overflowing bath.

Another approach to the problem of the overflowing bath will focus on the amount of water flowing into the bath and the number of pipes directing water into the tub. In other words, the causes of the problem rather than the symptoms. The solutions offered by these methods include removing some of the pipes altogether and turning down the flow on others. The overall result is to reduce the total load flowing into the bath so that it no longer overflows.

This handbook describes some of the food stressors which are found in most people's daily diets and suggests ways of either removing them or reducing them. As far as explaining mental and emotional health is concerned, food cannot be the whole picture but it is an important piece of the jigsaw. Food certainly does play a part in contributing to the total load which has been described as flowing into the bath.

As time goes by we are likely to discover the mental and emotional effects of stressors already known to cause physical problems in the body. These stressors can include environmental toxins such as chemical fertilizers, pesticides, herbicides, additives, antibiotics, growth promoters and pollutants (such as heavy metals, xenoestrogens, PCBs, dioxins). There are also certain naturally-occurring chemicals, micro-organisms (such as bacteria and viruses), mycotoxins (such as fungi) and parasites which can also pose hazards to health. In addition, a relatively recent potential risk to health of great concern to many people is the increasing presence of genetically modified organisms (GMOs) in the foods we buy.

Before we look at the specific signs and symptoms we might be experiencing from certain foods, we will first consider how the body manages to cope with an ever-increasing total load.

Remember that first strong cup of coffee, pint of beer or plate of cream cakes? Your body knows what's good for it and what isn't.

A Story of Stress

One way of describing how we cope is by telling a well-known story of stress, otherwise known as the General Adaptation Syndrome, originally penned by Professor Hans Selye back in the 1950s. There are four main chapters to this story and it is a tale that almost takes you full circle, back to where you started. But not quite, as you shall see.

CHAPTER ONE: ALARM BELLS

The Story of Stress begins – quite predictably – when your body first encounters something stressful. This can be anything, but we shall stick with food and drink. Remember that first strong cup of coffee, pint of beer or plate of cream cakes? Your body knows what's good for it and what isn't and, if you listen, this is when it will tell you. Your bodily alarm bells start to ring. Your heart may start beating faster than normal, you may get a headache or you may feel nauseous. Quite a dramatic start to the story, and it should have got your full attention. But unless a food or drink has a particularly unpleasant and dramatic effect, these symptoms may not be enough to prevent you from having more of it – particularly if you enjoyed the taste!

CHAPTER TWO: ALL ABOUT ADAPTATION

As we have seen with the bath, most people can cope with a certain amount of stress for a reasonable length of time without any difficulty. So, what happens next is that you may be pleasantly surprised. Even though you continue having the food or drink that produced such an initial shock to the system, you will find that the unpleasant symptoms have gone away! Because you are reasonably healthy, what has happened is that the body has been able to adapt to the alcohol/caffeine/cream cakes or whatever it was that initially 'disagreed' with you. The 'alarm' response the body initially produced when it was first exposed to the 'stressor' has disappeared. All is quiet on the symptom front. At least, for a while...

CHAPTER THREE: EXHAUSTION

Although things seem to be ticking along quite smoothly front of house, there is plenty of adapting going on backstage. And this costs energy. Energy which eventually starts to run low. Just as the annoying squeak or rattle on a car can portend a bigger problem down the road, your body produces early-warning signs that show you are beginning to run out of the ability to adapt to the stressors in your life. Low energy, low enthusiasm, low mood are all signs that your energy levels are running low. Physical aches and pains soon follow, coughs and colds, bloating, constipation, headaches and many of the other niggles that many of us may take as part-and-parcel of normal, modern life. The 'bath' is starting to overflow.

Now, the question that needs to be considered is this: do you take another painkiller and press on for another mile? Or do you slow down, maybe pull over to the side for a while and see if you can fix the problem before it becomes something much worse? If you choose to ignore the flashing fuel light that says you're getting low in petrol, sooner or later the car will come spluttering to a standstill. Human bodies can feel just like a car that's run out of fuel when exhaustion finally hits. Now you have no choice but to stop until you can recover your lost 'adaptive' energy.

CHAPTER FOUR: RECOVERY

When you're finally forced to your sick bed, it's unlikely that you'll have much of an appetite for the foods and drinks that may have contributed to your being there in the first place. And this is just as well because the key to your recovery will be to avoid (or at least reduce) the major stressors for just as long as it takes for your body to get back into balance again. Of course, if you've been sensible and heeded the early-warning signs, you'll probably have been able to stay out of bed. You may even have been able to keep your show on the road – perhaps by cutting down on the known stressors in your diet, maybe having them only 'once in a while'. Through making changes sooner rather than later you will have been able to sustain your ability to adapt to stress. You've been effectively managing your 'total load'.

THE FINAL CHAPTER: FULL CIRCLE?

Cutting out (or even just cutting down) the risky foods for a while (and substituting some things that are less harmful instead) reduced your total load. You are now feeling much better. With your experience of overdrawing on your 'adapting' reserves, you are now all too well aware of the negative effects too much of a food or drink can create for you. You have come full circle and are again aware of how food can make you feel.

EPILOGUE

Of course it's not quite back to where you started because you now know what happens if you overdo the alcohol, caffeine or cream cakes (or whatever your particular poisons are). Hopefully, you resist the temptation to overindulge in these foods and push on regardless until you hit the inevitable exhaustion stage. This time you manage things differently.

How this Handbook will Help

This handbook will guide you to manage your total load more effectively and enable you to continue coping with the remaining, and largely unavoidable, stressors of life. You will find out about the more common stressful foods. Some (probably unexpected) links between these foods and symptoms of emotional and mental ill health will be revealed. Where these foods can be found and where they are probably hidden in your daily diet will be shown to you. Whether you need to recover by cutting out certain foods completely or simply cut down on the amount of them that you eat, you will soon discover the tasty alternatives you can enjoy instead.

Good Mood Recipes

To introduce you to some of the foods recommended as beneficial for emotional and mental health, and also to give you an idea of alternatives you can substitute for some of the common culprit foods, *The Food and Mood Handbook* contains 10 Good Mood Recipes. These suggestions for good mood breakfasts, lunches, dinners and snacks can be found throughout the handbook and are excellent examples of quick and tasty, easy and economical dishes that should help you to feel good for longer.

The Good Mood Recipes are simple to make, so preparing and cooking them shouldn't add to your stress load. To help with food sensitivity investigations and rotation diet planning *(see relevant chapters of the handbook)*, each recipe has also been created to contain the maximum taste from the minimum number of ingredients. Reasons why these recipes are considered good for moods are summarized alongside the instructions, and fuller explanations can be found in the main body of the handbook. Enjoy!

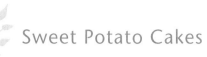

Sweet Potato Cakes

Type:	Snack
Equipment:	Oven
Preparation time:	10 mins
Cooking time:	30 mins

The natural sweetness of these savoury foods combine with the apple to produce a tasty and filling sweet snack. Sweet potatoes belong to a different food family from the more familiar white-fleshed potato (which is a member of the nightshade family). They contain antioxidant nutrients and have a lower Glycaemic Index than regular potatoes. Despite the name, buckwheat is no relation to wheat; instead it is in the same food family as rhubarb. It does not contain gluten and so makes a safe alternative for those sensitive to gluten-containing grains. Buckwheat is also rich in antioxidant bioflavonoids and minerals and has a low GI. The combination of sweet potato and buckwheat makes for a very slow energy-releasing snack.

Ingredients (serves 4)

200g/8oz/2 cups sweet potato, cooked with skin removed
100g/4oz/1 cup buckwheat flour
100g/4oz/1 cup milk-/dairy-free margarine
1 apple, chopped small
1 tsp chopped ginger
pinch cinnamon (optional)

Method

1   Preheat the oven to 200°C/375°F/Gas Mark 5.
2   Combine the ingredients in a bowl.
3   Form into four medium-sized or eight small balls, place onto a greased baking sheet and flatten slightly.
4   Bake for 30 mins.
5   Delicious eaten whilst still warm.

Ready?   Sticking a clean knife into the centre of the 'cakes' is a good
                  way to test whether or not they are ready.
Underdone   Knife comes out very sticky, and outside no darker in colour.
Just right   Knife comes out virtually clean, and outside slightly brown.
Overdone   Knife comes out clean, cake feels hard and outside is beginning
                  to burn.

Trouble-shooting tip   This recipe is so easy it is hard to imagine how it could go
                       wrong!

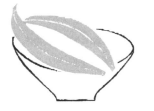

2
Craving Balance

So great is the power of some foods that it can be difficult, if not impossible, to resist the urge to eat them. Whether the desire is for a packet of biscuits, chunks of bread or lumps of cheese, sometimes it seems that the only way a craving can be silenced is for it to be satisfied.

Sometimes the need to eat or drink seems more than just a desire to satisfy hunger or thirst.

If only it were possible to eat when hungry and drink when thirsty and forget about food in between times. Unfortunately, the relationship with food is not always so straightforward. Sometimes the need to eat or drink seems more than just a desire to satisfy hunger or thirst. When a craving refuses to be silenced it can feel like it is the food that is in control of our thoughts or actions.

The trick is to find out what the cravings are telling us.

What we need to eat to stay well is determined by our genetic inheritance and our unique structure and functioning – the way our bodies are made and work. Also influencing what we eat are thoughts and emotions, and how we are used to behaving in certain situations. If these things somehow get out of balance, then cravings can start to become a problem. There are usually good reasons for food cravings. It can be the body's way of trying to keep itself in, or regain, balance. The trick is to find out what the cravings are telling us.

This handbook contains some ideas for understanding and coping with cravings. The next chapter will provide some information on how increased levels of certain brain chemicals, which can result from eating some foods, may actually reward the pleasure-centres of the brain. Brain chemistry can reinforce our eating behaviour so that we are more likely to continue eating a food. In Chapter 7 ('Caffeine and Chocolate'), the idea of addictive foods and drinks is revisited, describing how once we have become used to having something we can feel much worse if we stop. In the meantime, this chapter considers cravings as being a symptom of an imbalance of some sort, an unhealthy state which the body is attempting to correct.

Nutrient Needs

A craving could be a genuine need for a micronutrient such as a vitamin, mineral or essential fat.

Strong desires to eat or drink a specific food or beverage may be the body's way of telling us we need certain nutrients, that we are dehydrated – or both. A craving could be a genuine need for a micronutrient such as a vitamin, mineral or essential fat. Pregnant women, for example, can experience strong desires for strange combinations of food or even non-food substances such as dirt or chalk. Cravings for non-food substances is known as 'pica' and can also be experienced in some forms of mental illness. Pica can occur with certain nutritional deficiency states and is the body attempting to correct low levels of nutrients.

Overwhelming cravings for chocolate are experienced by many women only at a particular time of their menstrual cycle (often just before their period) and may indicate a physical requirement for particular nutrients readily available in chocolate which are needed more at the time of menstruation. For example, chocolate is a good source of iron and this mineral is a vital component of blood. Magnesium, particularly high in dark chocolate, is needed for (amongst other things) muscle contraction and relaxation. Craving chocolate at this time could be the body trying to satisfy an increased need for these nutrients in the only way it knows how.

Cravings for sugary or starchy foods such as sweets, biscuits, bread or pasta can also signal an urgent need for easily available energy or to raise levels of the brain chemical serotonin.

Cravings for sugary or starchy foods such as sweets, biscuits, bread or pasta can also signal an urgent need for easily available energy or to raise levels of the brain chemical serotonin. The chocolate cravings case study in this chapter describes how Barbara was able to bring her addiction to chocolate (which led her to consume up to six bars nearly every day) back under control. This craving was conquered by approaching the problem of chocolate cravings from the point of view of ensuring the body had a steady supply of energy. By successfully managing to 'even out' the highs and lows in her blood sugar levels, Barbara was able to resist the temptation to eat chocolate. Full details of the methods Barbara was able to use so successfully are given in Chapter 8. More information on serotonin can be found in Chapter 3.

Anatomy of a Chocolate Craving

People have been trying to explain the power of chocolate probably for as long as there has been chocolate to enjoy. The answer is likely to be a combination of physical factors and emotional associations. Some nutritional explanations for the appeal of a milk chocolate bar are offered below.

Ingredient	Why you might crave it
cocoa	– contains methylxanthines including theobromine and caffeine which have a stimulatory effect on the central nervous system
	– contains phenylethylamine which can raise levels of pleasure-giving endorphins in the brain
	– contains iron needed for blood formation
	– contains magnesium needed for the nervous system and muscle contraction and relaxation
	– contains fat which contributes to the pleasurable 'mouth feel' of chocolate
	– we may have evolved to experience fat as a highly desirable food for the energy it can provide in times of famine
milk	– a sensitivity to milk can give rise to cravings for milk
	– contains tryptophan which is converted to serotonin in the brain
sugar	– provides a quick fix for the symptoms of low blood sugar (such as low energy and mood), although there is often a price to be paid later on; helps with the absorption of tryptophan into the brain

Case Study: Cravings

Barbara (not her real name), a 25-year-old single parent, balancing the demands of young children and a university course, had ME/CFS (chronic fatigue syndrome). As is often the case with ME/CFS, Barbara was suffering from a variety of symptoms including fatigue, insomnia and poor quality sleep, memory difficulties and poor concentration. She frequently felt nauseous and suffered from food cravings, particularly for sweets or chocolate.

At her first appointment, Barbara admitted to consuming at least six bars of chocolate nearly every day. She was keen for this to change but wasn't sure how she would manage without her daily sugar and chocolate 'fixes'. It was explained that cravings for chocolate can be helped by regularly eating slow energy-releasing foods and in particular by not skipping breakfast. Cutting down on stimulant drinks such as tea and coffee at the same time can also make it much easier to resist temptation. Barbara agreed to these changes and planned to carry around with her some healthier snacks such as dried fruit, nuts, seeds and oatcakes to nibble on whenever she felt the urge.

Two weeks later, Barbara was feeling very pleased with herself. She reported that her consumption of chocolate had fallen from the usual 30 bars she would normally eat over this time to just six bars over the 14 days. Barbara explained that she had 'negotiated with herself' and the six bars had been rewards 'for not having so much chocolate' and that 'it helped to give in occasionally'. One of the most difficult times for Barbara had been when sitting with friends in the canteen at university and coping with the temptations of the vending machine. Temptation had been overcome through her determination together with a bag of tasty alternative nibbles which were always on hand to give her the 'oral gratification' she needed. Barbara explained that carrying around substitute snacks was her 'safety blanket' which prevented anxieties which could arise from her 'fear of being hungry'.

The changes Barbara had made were being helped by her not skipping breakfast and also by her cutting out the two cups of tea she was used to having each day. Although two cups is not, generally speaking, a high amount, Barbara's sensitivity to the tea was sufficiently great for her to soon notice a benefit from this change. Barbara found that she didn't miss her cuppas or her chocolate and at the same time she was 'noticing the sweetness and the tastes of food'. Barbara said she was now 'reading her energy levels' much more accurately, something she felt was essential for managing her lifestyle and her illness.

During the next two weeks, Barbara was able to gain even more control over her chocolate eating, eating only three bars over the 14 days. She then decided she had reached an acceptable level of chocolate consumption. When she did decide to treat herself she said she could now afford to buy the expensive, high-quality chocolate which did not make her feel nauseous. Eating regularly and finding and enjoying healthier alternative snacks had been crucial to her success. Barbara concludes: 'I can't believe the changes that have occurred in my health since I've made just a few simple adjustments to my diet. I feel like I'm more in control of what I eat instead of giving in to unhealthy cravings. In fact, I can't even stand chocolate most of the time. It's like I've re-programmed my brain.'

The Need for Balance

The idea of health as being a matter of balance is central to many systems of medicine. The term 'homeostasis' is used by orthodox and complementary practitioners alike to describe the body's in-built checks and balances that aim to keep things running smoothly. Whether or not we fully comprehend the mechanisms involved, it is becoming clearer how food has an important part to play in maintaining, or undermining, the functioning of mind and body.

Different medical systems use different models to describe and explain the idea of balance. When applied to the food we eat, each system offers an insight into what we could eat more of, and what we may need to eat less of, in order to feel well. All approaches to nutrition appear to start by grouping foods in one way or another. Problems are then associated with either too much, or not enough, of one or other category of food. Solutions are suggested which require a change in the balance of foods eaten. Ideally, individual characteristics are also recognized and accommodated by adjusting the combination of foods suggested.

Most of us are familiar with the idea of eating a 'balanced diet' and of the need to eat a variety of different foods to help us become – or remain – healthy. This idea of balance can vary between cultures but, whichever way we choose to view foods, all approaches have something to offer our understanding of the relationship between food and mood.

In the west we are used to thinking of foods as being divided up into protein foods (such as meat, fish, beans, cheese, eggs), carbohydrates (such as bread, pasta, potatoes, cakes, biscuits) and fatty foods (such as butter, cream and oils). In practice, a complete and largely unrefined food is likely to contain some protein, carbohydrate and fat, although one of these substances probably predominates. The protein, carbohydrate and fat groupings relate to how these food components are used by the body. More information on their relationship with the brain can be found in Chapter 10.

Eastern systems of medicine and philosophy divide foods according to the subtle effects they have on mind and body.

More common to eastern systems of medicine and philosophy are ideas of dividing foods according to the range of subtle effects they can have on mind and body. These approaches to food may use terms in pairs of opposites, such as the 'yin' and 'yang' of macrobiotics, or have groupings such as the three 'doshas' of Ayurvedic medicine or the five 'phases' of Oriental medicine.

Yin and Yang – Foods and Feelings

Different mental states can be supported or rebalanced by eating to regain a yin–yang balance.

Based on the work of the Japanese teacher George Oshawa, the macrobiotic system classifies foods into those that are, relatively speaking, more 'yin' or more 'yang'. Yin or yang are names given to the effect that eating these foods creates in the mind and body. Eating too much of either yin or yang foods can lead to a craving for those foods that have the opposite effect. For example, an excess of very yang foods such as meat, eggs, cheese and salt, can cause cravings for very yin foods such as alcohol, juices, coffee and sugar, in an attempt to regain a balance. Eating more of the 'balanced' foods (which have more or less equal yin and yang effects) such as wholegrains, beans, fruit and vegetables, nuts and seeds, can keep cravings under control.

Different mental states can be supported or rebalanced, according to this theory, by

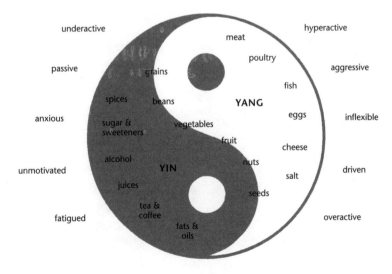

Fig 4 – The Yin and Yang of Food and Feelings

eating to regain a yin–yang balance. For example, a 'yin', anxious mental state which has been caused by eating too many sugary foods can be brought back into balance by eating more salty 'yang' foods. Impatience and 'driven' behaviour caused by a lot of animal protein, considered to be 'yang', may improve on having very 'yin' foods, such as fruit juices or sweet tea or coffee.

Five Phases of Foods and Feelings

One way to avoid an imbalance is to eat as varied a diet as possible.

A different and more complicated way of thinking about balance is the Oriental Theory of the Five 'Elements' or Five 'Phases'. It is based on the idea that life energy moves in specific predictable cycles. Each phase in the cycle influences the others and has traditional associations such as body organ, flavour sensation, type of food and mood. Energy imbalances in this system can show up as cravings for unusual combinations of foods. One way to avoid an imbalance, according to this theory, is to eat as varied a diet as possible. Use the diagram below to find out if any imbalances in your diet can be linked with any of the associated feelings.

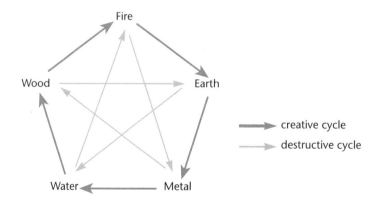

Phase	Fire	Earth	Metal	Water	Wood
Flavour	bitter	sweet	spicy	salty	sour
Food	stimulants	sweet food	protein food	salty food	fatty food
Feeling	anxious	worry	melancholy	fearful	angry

Fig 5 – Five Phases of Foods and Feelings

Oriental medicine also lists foods that are found to cause water retention or mucus formation. These foods are known as 'damp'-forming foods. The 'damp' foods correspond with many of the common culprit foods associated with emotional and mental symptoms. Particularly 'damp' foods include bananas, beer, milk and dairy products, oranges, peanuts, pork, saturated fats, sugar, tomatoes, wheat and yeast. Information on the link between food sensitivity and weight gain from water retention provoked by eating culprit foods can be found in Chapter 5.

Acidic and Alkaline Foods

Foods can also be classified as either acid-forming or alkalizing according to the effect they have on the body. This effect may be different to whether or not the food actually tastes acidic. For example, the acids of most fruits are metabolized to leave an alkaline 'ash' in the body and so are classed as alkaline foods. Both types of food are needed for balance, depending on individual metabolism, amount of physical activity and breathing pattern. It is generally easier to become over-acidic than over-alkaline so most people benefit from including a greater proportion of alkaline foods in their diet.

Cravings for alkalizing foods or drinks can indicate a need to redress an acid overload, which can be signalled by a range of symptoms which include poor concentration, insomnia, irritability and low libido. This imbalance may result from eating too many acid-forming sweets, cakes, fatty foods and meat. Fruit and vegetables and their juices can be eaten to redress the balance. An excess of alkalizing fruit or vegetables is less likely but it could create a need for acid-forming foods such as meat, fish, eggs or cheese.

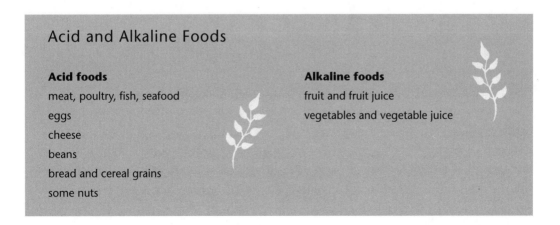

Acid and Alkaline Foods

Acid foods
meat, poultry, fish, seafood
eggs
cheese
beans
bread and cereal grains
some nuts

Alkaline foods
fruit and fruit juice
vegetables and vegetable juice

Using Test Strips to Measure pH

The pH of urine – which reflects the acid–alkali balance of blood and tissues – can be measured using test strips. Test strips can be obtained through a nutritional therapist and are a useful method of monitoring the effect of changes to your diet on your acid–alkali balance. A paper strip is held under the urine stream and then compared against a colour chart which indicates its acidity or alkalinity. Urine that is alkaline, with a pH value of 7 or more, is generally considered to be more healthy than urine that is more acidic.

Hyperventilation Syndrome

Over-alkalinity can be caused by chronic hyperventilation or 'over-breathing' which can create many of the symptoms that accompany food sensitivities. Emotional and mental symptoms caused by hyperventilation syndrome include anxiety, confusion, insomnia, nightmares, phobias, 'spacey' feeling, tension, lethargy, mood swings, visual hallucinations. An exercise for detecting this type of breathing pattern, and also one method for correcting it, can be found in Chapter 9. Some interesting facts about hyperventilation and the acid–alkali balance of the body are that:

- hyperventilation syndrome provokes the release of histamine which exaggerates allergic reactions
- deep sighing, which is common in habitual 'over-breathers', stimulates the release of endogenous opioids such as endorphins and counteracts depression
- foods can also affect breathing patterns, possibly due to their effect on the acid–alkali balance of the body chemistry
- extended vomiting, such as might occur in the eating disorder bulimia, can also cause a temporary over-alkaline state
- hyperventilation syndrome can also be associated with nutrient imbalances such as low levels of the mineral magnesium.

Food Plate

More familiar to the westerner is the idea of grouping foods to reflect the way most people shop for food and prepare meals. These food groups divide commonly-eaten foods into one of five different groups. These are:

- starchy staples (such as cereals, bread, pasta, potatoes)
- fruit and vegetables
- meat, fish and vegetarian substitutes
- dairy produce (such as milk, cheese and yoghurt)
- fatty and sweet and sugary foods (such as butter, cream, oils and crisps, cakes, sweets and biscuits).

The different food groups can then be shown in the form of a food 'plate' which is divided up to show the proportions recommended as being suitable for most adults and children over the age of two years. The food plate idea can be used for foods of other cultures and different diets without having to change the way the plate is divided up. A 'good mood' food 'plate' can be found in Chapter 11.

Exercise 3: What Do You Eat?

If you grouped together the main categories of food and drink that you usually consume and represented them as segments of a 'plate', what would the overall balance of your diet look like?

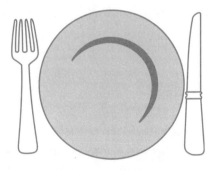

Fig 6 – Food plate

Understanding Cravings

Becoming more aware of the social and emotional triggers behind your impulses to eat can be a very useful first step to controlling unwanted cravings.

What you need to eat in order to feel good is different for everyone. Because you have a unique biochemistry, the foods that benefit you may not be as suitable for the next person. And individual needs can change also. A food that suits you today may not be what you need, or want, to eat tomorrow. Requirements for fuel and nutrients vary according to many factors which include the level of mental and physical activity, age, cycles of time such as the time of year or, for women, the 'time of the month'.

Environmental factors also have a part to play in determining what you should eat. Affecting your physical body will be the climate in which you live and whether you are spending your time indoors or outdoors, and also how hot or cold it is. Having an influence on your emotions at any one time will be factors such as the people you are with and what you are doing. Becoming more aware of the social and emotional triggers behind your impulses to eat can be a very useful first step to controlling unwanted cravings. Exercise 4 can help you to do this.

Exercise 4: Keeping a Food Triggers Diary

Choose a small notebook that you can carry around with you and write in discreetly. Use it to note down where you are, what you are doing and who you are with when you feel the urge to eat or drink something that, on reflection, you may wish you hadn't. When you look back at your notes, a pattern may be revealed that shows where and when you are at your most vulnerable. You can then start to think about how you could make changes to reduce the risk of succumbing to these unwanted food 'triggers'.

'Memory' Cravings

Cravings can apparently arise from the cleansing, or detoxifying, the body undergoes when changes are made to the diet. They occur as substances that have been stored in the body – maybe for years – are released back into the bloodstream to 'remind' the brain of previous foods encountered. These cravings can be for something familiar or which used to be eaten a lot. They usually disappear quite quickly. Otherwise, a 'memory craving' can be satisfied by eating or drinking just a small amount of the desired food. This should be sufficient to satisfy the craving until it disappears of its own accord.

Food that Satisfies

To manage food cravings it is helpful to eat food that both satisfies our immediate hunger and also provides sustained feelings of fullness.

Taste is most likely to influence what we choose to eat and the amount of fat, sugar or salt has an extremely powerful effect upon our enjoyment of a food. Not surprisingly, these ingredients are particularly high in much of the so-called 'junk food' burgers and biscuits that we generally love to eat. As described in Chapter 3, because of the way the appetite chemicals in our brain work, it is easy to eat too much fat or to get hooked on sugar.

To manage food cravings it is helpful to eat food that both satisfies our immediate hunger and also provides sustained feelings of fullness. One way of doing this is to choose foods that are digested slowly and release their energy over a longer time instead of foods that give a quick fix but don't satisfy for long. Chapter 8 provides useful information on how this can be done. Another guide to foods that satisfy is known as the Satiety Index.

Body, mind and food all work together to create sensations of nagging hunger followed by an experience of fullness and satisfaction after eating. If you think your cravings arise from genuine hunger pangs, it is worth paying attention to how well a food can fill you up, and how long it keeps you that way. According to the Satiety Index, foods that contain more protein, fibre and water and which have a lot of bulk will make you feel full for longer. Research has shown that potatoes are streets ahead for their ability to satisfy and fish is usually experienced as more filling (compared calorie for calorie) than either lean beef or chicken. Wholegrain bread is twice as filling as white bread and the satisfaction we can get from popcorn is apparently double that available from peanuts. Apples and oranges, as far as satiety is concerned, are apparently better than bananas.

The Satiety Index

This ranks foods on a scale according to their ability to satisfy hunger and stave off urges to eat again. Foods have been compared to white bread which was given a baseline score of 100 per cent. The higher the food's score on the Satiety Index, the better it is for filling you up and keeping you satisfied for longer. So far only a few foods have been tested but, according to research, 10 top foods to satisfy are:

Food	Score	Food	Score
Potatoes	323%	Baked beans	168%
Fish	225%	Wholemeal bread	157%
Porridge oats	209%	Popcorn	154%
Oranges	202%	Lentils	133%
Apples	197%	Brown rice	132%

So, why not start the day with a bowl of porridge or some wholemeal toast? Lunch could be a jacket potato with baked beans. Dinner could be rice with lentil curry and a fruit salad dessert. If you need something to eat between meal times you could do worse than choose popcorn which is a low-calorie, bulky and therefore satisfying snack.

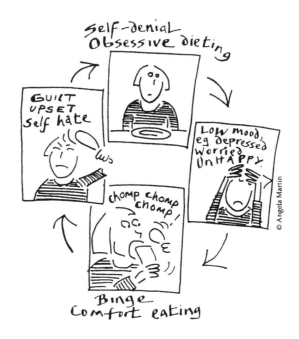

Carob Smoothie

Type:	Drink/Snack
Equipment:	blender
Preparation time:	3 mins
Cooking time:	none

Dedicated chocolate lovers can now enjoy a nutritious good mood chocolate-tasting treat. This smoothie – a drink or a light liquid snack – uses carob which is very similar to chocolate in taste but does not contain caffeine. The avocado creates a creamy texture and 'body', providing protein that includes the good mood nutrient tryptophan. It is also a good source of essential polyunsaturated oils and the antioxidant vitamin E. Avocados also contain good mood B-vitamins and potassium as well as many other vitamins and minerals. This needs to be prepared shortly before eating to maintain the fresh taste.

Ingredients (per person)

1 avocado
600ml/1 pint/2 cups rice milk (vanilla flavoured if available)
1 tbsp carob powder
1 tsp lemon juice (optional)

Method

1   Peel avocado and remove stone. Cut into small pieces.
2   Put all ingredients into blender and blend for approx. 1 min.
3   Pour into glasses and drink.
4   Use half the amount of rice milk to create a creamy dessert.

Trouble-shooting tip   Success is guaranteed with this recipe.

Having thought about how we could control cravings by creating a better balance in the diet, the next chapter looks at how the food we eat may actually affect the functioning of the brain.

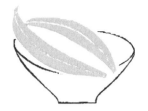

3

Brain Chemicals and Gut Feelings

It is possible to use the food–mood connection to help yourself towards better emotional and mental health. Although by no means the whole picture, the effects of food on mood are an important part of the mental health jigsaw. The puzzle that has to be pieced together to explain how food affects mood involves the brain, brain chemicals, and how these can be changed by what we eat.

Molecules of Emotions

Explanations into the effects of food on the emotions and the way the brain works focus on brain chemistry, for it is chemicals that make the connections between the network of neurons that make up the brain. As more brain chemicals are discovered there is speculation that different emotions are caused by different substances. Brain chemicals influence the way we think and feel and there are links between the type of foods that are eaten and the levels of certain chemical messengers, or neurotransmitters, in the brain. But instead of always locating particular thoughts, functions or feelings in specific places, the brain appears to function holistically as a complicated and coordinated network of activities. So, although there are brain chemicals and even 'molecules of emotion' which can be associated with different types of thinking and feeling, it seems unlikely that any one substance is entirely responsible for something as complex as a particular human emotion.

The separation between brain and body is an artificial distinction.

The Mind–Body Link

Mind–body (holistic) medicine has long held the view that the separation between brain and body is an artificial distinction, and the relatively new science of psychoneuroimmunology is now seeing the mind and immune system as interrelated. This means, for example, that emotions can affect the functioning of the immune system, a connection which is receiving attention in the treatment of certain illnesses such as cancer, and which gives rise to therapies such as meditation and visualization techniques to reduce the size of tumours. The idea of the mind and immune system being connected works both ways, so this approach to the body–mind may also explain why (for example) we can feel depressed when we're fighting off a cold or infection.

Brain Chemicals and Food

It appears that by choosing to eat certain foods the available amounts of some neurotransmitters can be altered.

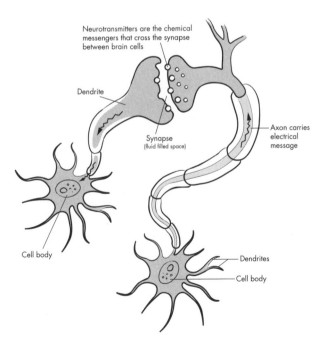

Neurotransmitters are the chemical messengers that cross the synapse between brain cells

Dendrite

Synapse (fluid filled space)

Axon carries electrical message

Cell body

Dendrites

Cell body

Fig 7 – Brain cells

Brain chemicals influence how we think, feel and behave, and the levels of some of these neuro-transmitters can be linked to what's been eaten. Although the relationship between food and mood-controlling brain chemicals is not fully understood, it appears that by choosing to eat certain foods the available amounts of some neurotransmitters can be altered. Examples of neurotransmitters that have been linked with the diet are serotonin (5-hydroxytryptamine), the catecholamines, dopamine and noradrenaline (norepinephrine), and also acetylcholine.

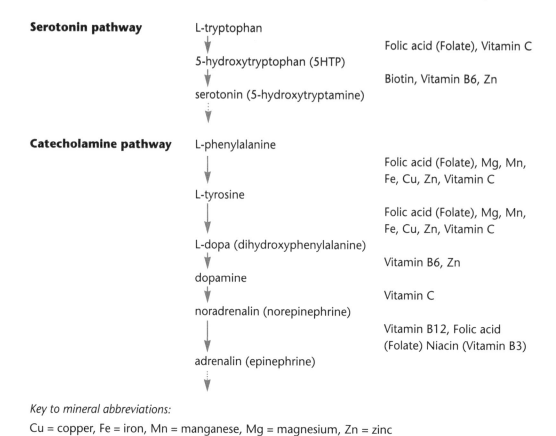

Serotonin pathway

L-tryptophan

Folic acid (Folate), Vitamin C

5-hydroxytryptophan (5HTP)

Biotin, Vitamin B6, Zn

serotonin (5-hydroxytryptamine)

Catecholamine pathway

L-phenylalanine

Folic acid (Folate), Mg, Mn, Fe, Cu, Zn, Vitamin C

L-tyrosine

Folic acid (Folate), Mg, Mn, Fe, Cu, Zn, Vitamin C

L-dopa (dihydroxyphenylalanine)

Vitamin B6, Zn

dopamine

Vitamin C

noradrenalin (norepinephrine)

Vitamin B12, Folic acid (Folate) Niacin (Vitamin B3)

adrenalin (epinephrine)

Key to mineral abbreviations:
Cu = copper, Fe = iron, Mn = manganese, Mg = magnesium, Zn = zinc

Fig 8 – Brain chemical 'pathways'

The life journey of a brain chemical is described as its 'metabolic pathway', and a brain chemical can have several 'identities' during its lifetime. Two important brain chemical pathways are shown above. The first describes the serotonin pathway and the second is the catecholamine pathway, which features the neurotransmitters dopamine and noradrenalin (norepinephrine). Both pathways start with the amino acids found in food, and each stage of the journey requires various co-factors (or helpers) which include vitamins and minerals. These pathways conclude with the breaking down or degradation of the neurotransmitters by enzymes such as monoamine oxidase (MAO) and catechol-o-methyltransferease (COMT).

Antidepressants

Most antidepressant medication has the effect of increasing the abnormally low levels of neurotransmitters understood to be associated with symptoms of depression. The neurotransmitters serotonin, dopamine and noradrenaline (norepinephrine) belong to a group of chemicals called monoamines. Levels of monoamines in the brain are controlled by various mechanisms including an enzyme called monoamine oxidase (MAO) which breaks down used or excess monoamines through a chemical process called oxidation.

One type of antidepressant medication known as monoamine oxidase inhibitors (MAOIs) works by inhibiting the action of MAO, thus allowing the 'excitatory' neurotransmitters to accumulate in the synapse and stimulate cell-to-cell communication. Other medications, such as the tricyclics and SSRIs (selective serotonin reuptake inhibitors), function in a slightly different way by preventing the reuptake of used neurotransmitters. A well-known example of a SSRI is Prozac (fluoxetine).

But whichever drug is used, the end result appears to be the same: increased levels of brain chemicals building up in the gap between brain cells. The effectiveness of the herb St John's Wort (*Hypericum perforatum*) in the treatment of depression has been explained by its ability to raise neurotransmitter levels using either (or both) of the mechanisms described above.

Serotonin for Relaxation

Eating tryptophan-containing foods is one way of potentially boosting brain serotonin levels.

Serotonin is a brain chemical associated with various moods and behaviours including reducing appetite and curbing impulses, enhancing mood and promoting sleep. Low levels of serotonin can be responsible for feelings of depression, and antidepressant medication often works by raising serotonin levels. Serotonin in the brain is made from tryptophan, an amino acid, or protein fragment, found in protein-containing foods. Therefore, eating tryptophan-containing foods is one way of potentially boosting brain serotonin levels.

However, the absorption of tryptophan across the blood–brain barrier into the brain where it can be converted into serotonin is helped by eating carbohydrate-rich foods. And because of the serotonin-enhancing effect of carbohydrate foods, many cravings for sugary or starchy snacks can be a subconscious attempt to correct the unpleasant symptoms of low serotonin levels in the brain. Your carbohydrate cravings (for sweet and starchy food such as biscuits, cake, bread, pasta) could be your body crying out for more serotonin.

What this means in practice is that, to get the full benefit of the tryptophan from the protein food you have eaten, you need to follow your tryptophan protein meal with a food that contains mostly carbohydrates. But, to avoid a roller-coaster sugar high followed by a low you need to take care with the type of carbohydrate you choose. Chapter 8 contains more information on the best carbohydrates to choose.

Because eating a carbohydrate-rich meal boosts sleep-promoting serotonin levels, having something starchy like pasta at lunchtime could prove counterproductive. If you want to stay alert during the afternoon, you need to increase levels of the brain chemicals that can help you to do this. So, if you find yourself needing an afternoon nap whilst you are still at work, then look at what you had for lunch.

Your carbohydrate cravings (for sweet and starchy food such as biscuits, cake, bread, pasta) could be your body crying out for more serotonin.

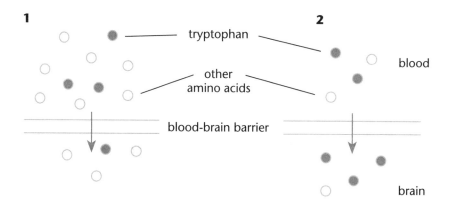

Fig 9 – Absorption of tryptophan

1   After eating protein, tryptophan is present in the blood but has to compete with other amino acids for absorption across the blood–brain barrier.

2   After eating carbohydrate, insulin is released which selectively binds with the other amino acids to transport them to muscles. However, tryptophan is not taken and is left behind at the blood–brain barrier. Without any competition, more tryptophan is able to cross into the central nervous system, where it can be converted into mood-enhancing serotonin.

Dopamine and Noradrenaline (Norepinephrine) for Action

During the day we are likely to need to stay awake, alert and active and the brain chemicals that help us do this include dopamine and noradrenaline (norepinephrine). Lower levels of dopamine and noradrenaline (norepinephrine) can result from low levels of the amino acids tyrosine and phenylalanine, which are needed to make these neurotransmitters. Low levels of tyrosine have been associated with depression where apathy and lack of motivation are key symptoms. Protein-rich foods which contain tyrosine and phenylalanine, such as meat, fish, beans, nuts, seeds, soya and cheese, are better suited to keeping up our levels of these neurotransmitters and can make better choices for foods to eat at lunchtime.

Protein-rich foods can make better choices for foods to eat at lunchtime.

Acetylcholine for Memory

Acetylcholine is associated with learning and memory function and is found to be low in cases of dementia such as Alzheimer's disease. Acetylcholine is formed from choline or lecithin (phosphatidylcholine) which is found in foods such as eggs, liver, brewer's yeast, meats, fish, soya beans, wheatgerm, corn and peanuts. However, the relationship between eating choline or lecithin-rich foods and levels of acetylcholine in the brain are not as clear as for other neurotransmitters. Phosphatidylcholine (lecithin) is a member of a group of fats known as phospholipids. Another well-known phospholipid is phosphatidylserine (PS).

Brain Chemicals and Food

Neurotransmitter:	serotonin
important for:	appetite control, mood and sleep
made from:	tryptophan, an amino acid found in protein foods which is carried into the brain in the presence of carbohydrates
some food sources:	poultry, oil-rich fish, beans, baked potatoes, oats, nuts and seeds *(Chapter 8 contains recommendations for carbohydrate foods which help the absorption of tryptophan)*
Neurotransmitters:	dopamine and noradrenaline (norepinephrine) are catecholamine neurotransmitters
important for:	staying awake, being alert and active
made from:	tyrosine and phenylalanine, amino acids found in protein
some food sources:	meat, fish, beans, nuts, seeds, soya and cheese
Neurotransmitter:	acetylcholine
important for:	memory and learning
made from:	choline (a fat-liking, vitamin-like substance) and lecithin (a phospholipid or type of fat)
some foods sources:	higher levels of choline and lecithin are found in eggs, liver, wheatgerm, brewer's yeast, fish, soya beans, corn and peanuts

Production of these neurotransmitters depends on vital co-factors (helping substances) which include vitamins and minerals. It is therefore important to eat a varied diet which contains plenty of fresh fruit and vegetables in order to obtain the nutrients your brain needs.

Endorphins

Levels of mood-altering endorphins can also be increased after eating certain foods and drinks. Endorphins are the body's own opium-like substances whose effects include feelings of euphoria, high self-esteem and a reduction in physical and emotional pain. They are well-known for creating what is called the 'runner's high' that can be experienced during strenuous exercise. However, the downside of eating foods that have an endorphin-raising effect is that, with repeated exposure to excessive amounts, they may result in an addictive relationship with the food. For example, the phenylethylamine in chocolate which is thought to raise endorphin levels may account for some of the very 'moreish' quality of chocolate.

Tryptophan-containing Foods

Tryptophan is just one of eight 'essential' amino acids (protein building blocks) that cannot be made by the body and which have to be obtained from food in relatively balanced amounts. Some good sources of tryptophan, together with the approximate amounts present in common foods, are given below. The tryptophan content of foods varies and these figures represent typical levels present in an average-sized portion. The tryptophan-containing foods listed here are those less likely to be linked with food sensitivity reactions.

Food	Portion size	Amount of tryptophan per portion
chicken	100g/3¹/₂oz/¹/₂ cup	360mg
turkey	100g/3¹/₂oz/¹/₂ cup	340mg
tuna	85g/3oz/¹/₂ cup	280mg
salmon	85g/3oz/¹/₂ cup	260mg
kidney beans	170g/6oz/1 cup	180mg
rolled oats	85g/3oz/1 cup	175mg
lentils	200g/7oz/1 cup	160mg
chickpeas	200g/7oz/1 cup	140mg
pumpkin seeds	30g/1oz/¹/₄ cup	120mg
sunflower seeds	30g/1oz/¹/₄ cup	100mg
baked potato with skin	1 large	75mg
tahini (sesame butter)	1 tablespoon	56mg
walnuts	25g/1oz/¹/₃ cup	50mg
avocado	1 medium	40mg
almond butter	1 tablespoon	40mg

SAD?

Seasonal Affective Disorder (SAD) is associated with symptoms of depression, lethargy, loss of libido and cravings for carbohydrate foods to raise low serotonin levels. Low serotonin levels found in SAD sufferers may be due to a hormone imbalance and the effect of higher than normal levels of the hormone melatonin.

Melatonin is a hormone made from tryptophan via serotonin and its is important for mood and sleep–wake cycles. Secreted by the pineal gland, the amount released is related to the amount of darkness in a 24-hour period. The longer the night, the more melatonin is released as we are naturally encouraged by this circadian rhythm to sleep when the sun goes down. Light falling on the retina of the eye reduces the amount of serotonin that is converted to melatonin which is why many SAD sufferers benefit from using light boxes to create artificial daylight.

Histamine

Histamine is an important brain chemical involved in the immune system and allergic reactions. Both excessively high and abnormally low levels of histamine have been associated with mental health problems. Symptoms of excessive histamine (histadelia) have been linked with abnormal fears, addictions, 'blank mind', compulsive behaviour, confusion, depression, emotional instability, hyperactivity, insomnia, obsessions, schizophrenia, suicide, thought disorders. Low levels of histamine (histapenia) have been found in people suffering with anxiety, hallucinations, paranoia and schizophrenia.

The genetic predisposition to abnormal histamine levels has also been linked with imbalances in levels of important vitamins and minerals. Histamine is made in the body from histidine, an amino acid found in protein foods. Histamine levels may be affected by certain foods which contain naturally-occurring histamine or which may stimulate the release of histamine in the body. Some of these foods are listed in Chapter 6 in the section on naturally-occurring amines.

Creamy Turkey or Chicken Rainbow Salad

Type: Lunch/Dinner
Equipment: Blender (for almond 'cream')
Preparation time: 10 mins
Cooking time: None (use precooked turkey/chicken)

Turkey and chicken are excellent sources of tryptophan protein which is eventually converted in the brain to the relaxing neurotransmitter serotonin. In the meantime, if you tend to suffer from mid-afternoon slumps in energy, having a protein-based lunch such as this can provide the solution. The almond 'cream' is so easy to make and provides the texture that turns this dish into a special treat. This method can be used to make other nut or seed 'creams' or 'milks' – try cashew nuts as an alternative to almonds in this recipe. Different natural colours in fruits and vegetables indicate the presence of beneficial brain-protecting antioxidant phytochemicals. Choose a range of vegetables giving a rainbow of colours to ensure the broadest possible protection from these vital nutrients.

Ingredients (per person)

100g/4oz/1 cup cooked turkey/chicken
red-coloured vegetable e.g. ¼ red pepper or one large tomato
orange-coloured vegetable e.g. 1 carrot
yellow-coloured vegetable e.g. ¼ yellow pepper or 50g/2oz/¼ cup sweet corn
green-coloured vegetable or herb e.g. handful of watercress
30g/1oz/¼ cup almonds
60ml/2fl oz/¼ cup water

Method

1   Cut the chicken into small pieces.
2   Chop the vegetables into small pieces.
3   Blend almonds with enough water to make a creamy paste.
4   Combine all ingredients in a bowl and serve.

Brain Regulation

The brain does its best to prevent levels of neurotransmitters from becoming too high or falling too low so that it does not become over- or under-stimulated as a consequence. To maintain a happy medium the brain can usually 'turn up' or 'turn down' the volume of communication between its neurons and regulate the amount of chemical messengers received and electrical messages transmitted. One way of doing this is to vary the number of 'receptors' that are available to welcome a particular type of neurotransmitter after it has crossed the gap between brain cells.

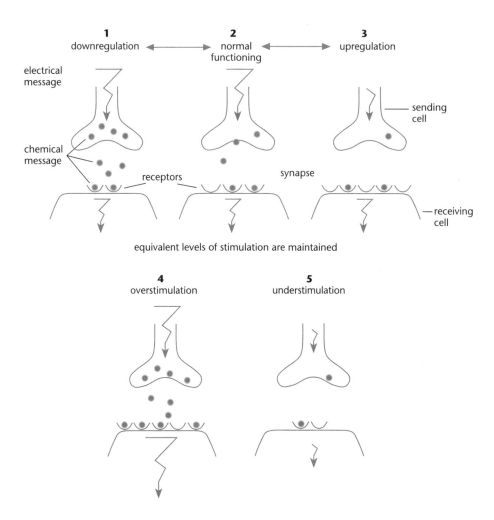

Fig 10 – Brain balancing

Increasing the numbers of available receptors can compensate for lower levels of a brain chemical and may occur in some people with a tendency to low levels of certain neurotransmitters. This is known as 'upregulating' and it is about making the best of low levels of a neurotransmitter. Higher levels of brain chemicals can be balanced by 'down-regulating', or reducing, the number of receptors available. In this way the brain can control, to a certain degree, the level of chemical messages that are received and electrical messages transmitted. Neurons can avoid being over- or under-stimulated and the brain can stay in balance.

Addiction and Withdrawal

If a receiving cell is exposed to an unusually large quantity of brain chemical (such as an endorphin-like substance originating from within the body) or chemical (such as a drug) that originates from outside the body, the excessive stimulation can be experienced as a pleasant 'high'.

If regularly experienced, the overwhelming, pleasurable sensation may become difficult to repeat because, in anticipation of more of the chemical, the brain can respond by 'up-regulating' its response. This is when more receptors for a substance are made available to cope with the increased supplies that are now expected. When this happens the brain is ready and waiting for more of the same highly stimulating experience.

Certain foods such as chocolate and sugar are thought to increase levels of the pleasure-giving endorphins in the brain.

Brain regulation can be used to explain the apparently addictive nature of some foods and drinks. For example, certain foods such as chocolate, sugar or even peptides formed from the incomplete digestion of gluten or casein protein (*see later section*), are thought to increase levels of the pleasure-giving endorphins in the brain. If supplies of these foods are regular, then the brain can 'up-regulate' itself and increase the number of endorphin receptors available. The result is that more and more of the food appears to be needed to create the same overwhelming pleasurable effect first experienced.

Unfortunately, 'just saying no' to a food is not always that straightforward.

Chasing the initial high produced by a substance soon becomes ineffective but, unfortunately, 'just saying no' to a food is not always that straightforward. Although a high may no longer be experienced from having a food or beverage, if regular doses of it are stopped altogether then the upregulated brain receptors are left 'unsatisfied' and waiting for a 'hit' that never comes. This situation can be associated with unpleasant 'withdrawal symptoms'.

Any unpleasant symptoms that improve upon consuming a food or beverage are a sure sign that the body has become 'hooked' on a substance and is starting to complain when it is withdrawn. The start–stop, pleasure and pain, of binge or comfort eating may be linked to experiencing the highs and lows – too much and then not enough – of certain brain chemicals. As with any drug, it is wise to make slow and gradual changes to minimize the discomfort of withdrawal.

Withdrawal symptoms diminish as the brain readjusts itself once more. This time the brain 'downregulates' and reduces the number of receptors available for that chemical effect. If the changes are maintained and less – rather than more – of the 'addictive' substance is forthcoming, then a calmer state of balance is eventually regained.

If the changes are maintained, then a calmer state of balance is eventually regained.

Gut Feelings

'The primary seat of insanity generally is in the region of the stomach and intestines', said Pinel, a French psychiatrist, in 1807, who obviously recognized the importance of the gut in emotional and mental health. Yet precisely how and why the gut is important to the health of the brain is only just beginning to be understood.

The nervous system, which sends and receives messages that influence the way the body functions, has nerve fibres extending throughout the body. It is masterminded by the brain and spinal cord, known as the central nervous system, which in turn controls the peripheral nervous system. The idea that the brain in your head is not the only physical location of the mind can be useful for our exploration into food and mood.

The gut can be seen as an extension of the brain.

Brain chemicals or 'informational substances' associated with different mental and emotional states can also be found in the digestive system. Special receptors which join up with particular brain chemicals have been found situated in the gut. This means that the gut can be seen, in this respect, as an extension of the brain. This finding goes some way to explain familiar 'gut feelings' or the sensation that emotions are felt in the abdominal area.

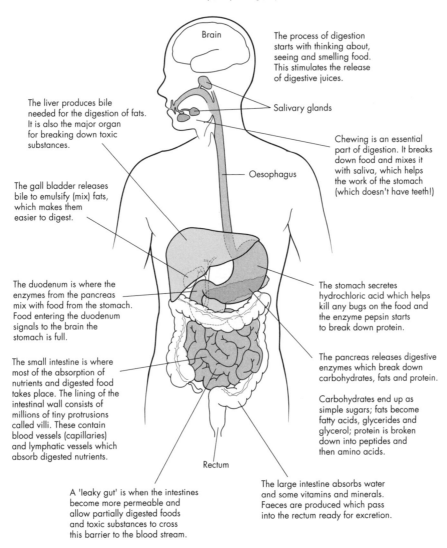

The journey from top to bottom can take from a few hours to a few days, depending on your diet

Brain

The process of digestion starts with thinking about, seeing and smelling food. This stimulates the release of digestive juices.

The liver produces bile needed for the digestion of fats. It is also the major organ for breaking down toxic substances.

Salivary glands

Chewing is an essential part of digestion. It breaks down food and mixes it with saliva, which helps the work of the stomach (which doesn't have teeth!)

The gall bladder releases bile to emulsify (mix) fats, which makes them easier to digest.

Oesophagus

The duodenum is where the enzymes from the pancreas mix with food from the stomach. Food entering the duodenum signals to the brain the stomach is full.

The stomach secretes hydrochloric acid which helps kill any bugs on the food and the enzyme pepsin starts to break down protein.

The small intestine is where most of the absorption of nutrients and digested food takes place. The lining of the intestinal wall consists of millions of tiny protrusions called villi. These contain blood vessels (capillaries) and lymphatic vessels which absorb digested nutrients.

The pancreas releases digestive enzymes which break down carbohydrates, fats and protein.

Carbohydrates end up as simple sugars; fats become fatty acids, glycerides and glycerol; protein is broken down into peptides and then amino acids.

Rectum

A 'leaky gut' is when the intestines become more permeable and allow partially digested foods and toxic substances to cross this barrier to the blood stream.

The large intestine absorbs water and some vitamins and minerals. Faeces are produced which pass into the rectum ready for excretion.

Fig 11 – Digestion Journey

Leaky Gut and Leaky Brain

In a healthy body, most food is completely digested before it passes through the gut lining and into the bloodstream. For some people, though, the enzyme mechanism responsible for breaking down food appears to be faulty in some way. This means that larger than normal amounts of incompletely-digested food can end up passing through the gut lining to be circulated around the body in the bloodstream. Another reason suggested for the higher than average amounts of partially digested food particles getting into the blood is that the gut lining in some people has become, literally, 'leaky'. Otherwise known as 'intestinal permeability', this is when the gut lining becomes more porous to allow greater quantities of abnormally large molecules to enter the bloodstream and circulate throughout the body.

Intestinal Hyperpermeability

Intestinal hyperpermeability is now being linked with many conditions including autism, multiple food sensitivities and chronic fatigue syndrome. A suspected 'leaky gut' may be diagnosed by a special urine test called the 'lactulose-mannitol challenge' which is available through nutritional therapists. The causes of gut permeability are uncertain and may include a genetic predisposition in combination with physical damage from surgery, damage which may arise from chemicals, excessive alcohol or the effects of an infection, parasites or gut dysbiosis (imbalance of intestinal flora).

Once absorbed into the bloodstream, the components of digested food are circulated around the body as nutrients for the various cells and tissues. On the journey around the body the nutrients in the blood travel to the brain. Here, the contents of the blood are separated from the cells of the brain by a barrier, aptly named the blood–brain barrier. The blood–brain barrier is made up of a layer of tightly-packed cells whose job it is to stop unwanted substances such as certain chemicals, drugs or viruses from entering the brain. For reasons yet to be understood, in some people the blood–brain barrier appears to be less effective at keeping out substances such as partially digested food components which can then enter the central nervous system and disrupt the normal functioning of the brain.

Healthy Bowels, Healthy Brain

Chronic constipation can lead to increased levels of toxins circulating in the blood which can also impact on brain functioning.

As we have seen, the state of your mind is likely to be linked to the state of your bowels, as many brain-influencing chemicals are also found in the gut. Chronic constipation can lead to increased levels of toxins circulating in the blood which can also impact on brain functioning. If you would like to make sure your gut feelings are good ones, take note of the following suggestions for keeping a healthy digestive system.

- Eat plenty of fresh fruit and vegetables to 'keep you regular'. The minimum recommended amount for an adult is about 400g or five 80g portions of fruits and vegetables every day. If you don't have kitchen scales handy, then a portion can be thought of as about a handful. The 'five-a-day' doesn't include protein-rich nuts or starchy, carbohydrate-rich vegetables such as potatoes. Fresh fruit or vegetable juices can only count towards one of the five recommended portions.
- Drink lots of water every day. Constipation may simply be a matter of dehydration. Aim for about 2 litres or 8 glasses of plain water. Water is also recommended as an essential good mood nutrient – turn to Chapter 10 for more information.
- Include fibre-containing foods in your daily diet. Apart from the fruit and vegetables mentioned above, fibre-providers include wholegrains such as wholemeal bread and pasta, brown rice, beans, peas and lentils and bran. Bran can be added to foods to increase the fibre content of a meal. Oat and rice bran are less likely to irritate the gut lining of sensitive people.
- Eat linseeds. Apart from containing valuable essential fatty acids, these seeds can be used whole as a food that swells to increase the size of stools and help with constipation. To have this effect the seeds need to be taken with lots of liquid. Linseeds can be used in many ways in cooking and baking; they can be sprinkled onto foods or added to porridge or soups.
- Reduce the risk of gut dysbiosis which is an imbalance in the bowel 'flora' – naturally-occurring yeasts and bacteria in the gut. For example, an excessive yeast or candida overgrowth in the gut can be associated with symptoms of depression, poor concentration and fatigue. Cutting down on concentrated sugars is an important first step. A yeast sensitivity is often associated with this condition and so having less yeast-containing food, particularly leavened bread, wine and beer, can also help. Dysbiosis in the gut takes time to correct and the support of a nutritional therapist is recommended. She (or he) will be able to advise on the many dietary changes that can help. Foods, such as live yoghurt, and supplementation with antifungals, probiotics (such as *Lactobacillus acidophilus*) and prebiotics (such as fructo-oligosaccharides) to encourage the 'good' gut flora can also be beneficial.
- Heal a 'leaky gut' by avoiding or reducing alcohol which can increase intestinal permeability. Consult a nutritional therapist who can provide a laboratory test to assess gut permeability and advise on nutritional supplements to help remove unwanted microorganisms or parasites and support the gut healing process.

♣ Avoid any foods to which you are sensitive and which may be irritating to the gut lining. Chapter 5 has information on how to do this.

♣ Learn to cope with stress through, for example, breathing and relaxation techniques. The gut–brain connection works both ways and the state of your mind will affect the state of your digestive system *(Chapter 9 contains one example of a breathing exercise)*.

Time and Motion Studies

The time it takes for food to travel the long journey from the top to the bottom of the digestive system is known as the 'transit time'. It can be measured by eating something such as sweetcorn, beetroot, whole sesame seeds or whole linseeds (which tend to pass through undigested) and timing how long it takes to pass through. To measure your transit time, note when you eat the 'test food' and keep an eye on the contents of the toilet pan until the same food reappears. When it does appear, note how many hours have elapsed.

Each person's rate of digestion is different, but if your transit time is much more than 24–48 hours then you could be constipated. Consult the section above for the simple steps you can take to help with constipation and to generally improve the health of your gut.

Another measure of bowel health is the type of stool that you pass. Keeping an eye on the contents of the toilet pan will show how different foods are dealt with by your body. The ideal stool is one that

♣ is solid and not too 'loose' or runny
♣ comes out easily
♣ floats but breaks up on flushing the toilet
♣ is a mid-brown in colour
♣ is not too smelly
♣ consists of large pieces (rather than small 'rabbit droppings')
♣ does not contain any blood or mucus (it is particularly important that you consult your doctor if either of these symptoms are present).

Food Effects

Food and drink can have an apparently toxic effect on the brain and body due to some of the chemicals they contain. Artificial chemical additives, such as food colourings, can be one example but food contains natural substances which may also affect mood (*see Chapter 6*). And there are other mood-altering substances which can be created during the process of digestion that affect the functioning of the brain.

The effects on mood of some food appear to be related to partially-digested components of food circulating in the bloodstream and affecting the brain and central nervous system. For example, proteins from certain foods can be associated with an immune response that can be linked to a range of symptoms such as anxiety, depression or fatigue. This type of food sensitivity seems to involve an antibody known as immunoglobulin-G or 'IgG'. The immune response associated with these delayed or 'hidden' reactions to food is somewhat different to that associated with classical food allergies. Classical food allergies involve 'IgE' antibodies and tend to provoke immediate, obvious and sometimes very severe symptoms.

Food as a Drug

Opium-like peptides are thought to derive from partially-digested foods such as the gluten protein found in wheat and the milk protein (known as casein) found in milk and dairy produce.

The brain function of some susceptible people can be affected by certain abnormal protein fragments known as peptides. Peptides are made up of chains of amino acids and certain peptides appear, in some people, to be capable of producing a drug-like effect on the brain. The effect of these peptides can be comparable to that of opiate drugs such as heroin and morphine. The opium-like peptides arising from faulty digestion may derive from partially-digested foods such as the gluten protein found in wheat (also present in rye, barley and oats) and the milk protein (known as casein) found in milk and dairy produce.

The brain is able to respond to opioid (morphine-like) substances from food because it has special receptors ready to receive the body's own internally-made (endogenous) opioid chemicals such as the endorphins and enkaphalins.

Some foods such as chocolate, sugar and alcohol have an endorphin-raising effect which may be why these foods appear to be so addictive if consumed regularly and in large amounts.

A urine test is able to measure levels of a 'marker' substance called IAG (indolyl acryloyl glycine). IAG can result from faulty processing of tryptophan and has been linked with raised levels of the problem opioid peptides. People showing raised IAG in their urine usually then benefit from a gluten- and casein-free diet.

Are You Satisfied?

There are a number of neurotransmitters responsible for controlling appetite. Some increase the desire for food, others create a feeling of satisfaction and fullness. Endorphins, noradrenaline (norepinephrine) and neuropeptide Y all increase the appetite, whereas appetite-suppressing neurotransmitters include cholecystokinin (CCK), serotonin and corticotropin releasing factor, which all reduce the desire for food. Levels of circulating neurotransmitters can be influenced by various means including the amount of sex and exercise we have, breathing patterns, drugs and food. Some food-related influences on the appetite-controlling neurotransmitters are given opposite.

If you eat too fast and don't chew your food properly it is possible to overeat before the message that you are full gets through to the brain.

Chewing Things Over

The sense of satiety or feeling of fullness after a meal is controlled by a neurotransmitter hormone called cholecystokinin (CCK) which is released by the digestive system. This feedback mechanism takes time to work and if you eat too fast and don't chew your food properly it is possible to overeat before the message that you are full gets through to the brain. Also, if you are relying on your brain to tell you when to stop eating, it is easier to overindulge in fatty foods than to have too much carbohydrate. Remember, your stomach doesn't have teeth and needs you to chew your food well to release important nutrients from the food. The phrase 'chewing something over' in your mind to describe thinking something through may have a literal meaning as there is some evidence that the physical act of chewing improves memory!

Appetite, Brain Chemicals and Food

Neurotransmitters that raise appetite include:

endorphins — increased levels can result from eating chocolate, sugar, opioid peptides from faulty digestion of wheat or milk. Also sex, exercise, yogic breathing and meditation

noradrenaline (norepinephrine) — increased levels can result from eating protein (such as meat, fish, beans, nuts) and in particular foods containing tyrosine and phenylalanine (amino acid protein fragments)

neuropeptide Y — fasting or long gaps between meals and exercise all raise levels of this neurotransmitter

Neurotransmitters that reduce appetite include:

cholecystokinin (CCK) — increased levels of this neurotransmitter are triggered by food in the duodenum and give rise to a feeling of fullness after eating

serotonin — carbohydrates (starchy, sugary foods) raise levels of serotonin because of their ability to increase absorption of tryptophan. Tryptophan, an amino acid found in protein-containing food, is converted to serotonin in the brain. Some foods such as avocados, bananas, pineapples, plantain, plums, tomatoes and molluscs (such as octopus) contain significant amounts of ready-made serotonin

corticotropin releasing factor — this is released in response to stress. Stress reduces the effectiveness of the digestive system and also our desire to eat

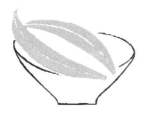

4

Symptoms
and Suspects

We have seen some of the ways food can affect how we feel. Now we need to find out which foods – if any – are the culprits, guilty of contributing to symptoms of ill health. But first, just how bad can some foods make us feel and which substances should we suspect?

You Are the Expert

You have a unique experience of the world inside and outside your physical body. Because everyone is different, a situation that is a source of stress for one person can be embraced and enjoyed by another. No-one but you can get inside your head, and only you can directly experience your emotions and thoughts. You may be surrounded by loving and supportive friends, family or work colleagues, but only you can know exactly how you feel and how you think. So, although other people's advice and opinions on your emotional and mental health can be extremely useful, only you can be the expert on your own mind.

A Label for How You Feel

Some uncomfortable emotional, mental and physical experiences can be seen as symptoms of underlying distress. They can be related to each other and recognized as a specific disease, illness or condition. The clustering of experiences into 'disease labels' can enable organizations to provide, and people to access, better health care. Other times a diagnosis is a hindrance in life, and may even carry a social stigma.

What you feel and how you behave is influenced by many things including where you live and the people around you. Feelings and behaviours that are considered acceptable or 'normal' within one family or culture may be judged as unacceptable or threatening if experienced or expressed within a different environment. So it is worth remembering that the degree to which you (and others) consider yourself as being healthy (or not) is likely to depend on the context in which you find yourself.

A food or beverage can change the way you behave and appear to others. The well-known influence of alcohol on the mind and body is one instance of this.

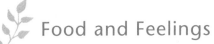

Food and Feelings

The intimate relationship you have with what you eat can provide many clues as to how food could be affecting your feelings. The consequences of consuming something may be experienced as largely physical; other influences of food and drink are more obviously emotional or mental. For example, a food or beverage can change the way you behave and appear to others. The well-known influence of alcohol on the mind and body is one instance of this; the 'buzz' available from a cup of coffee and the caffeine it contains is another. Then there are the foods and effects of food that are not so well known.

Listed below are some emotional and mental health difficulties and illnesses that may be made worse or which, in some cases, may even be caused, by foods or abnormal levels of certain nutrients. Because of the complexity of the food–mood relationship, and each person's unique biochemistry, it could be misleading to link particular foods with specific feelings. However, the breadth of food's potential influence on mood can be shown by the wide range of 'symptoms' that are listed. Some of the 'symptoms' are relatively minor in the disruption they can cause to daily life, but most of those listed will be considered problematic if experienced too often.

Symptoms

Food can be a crucial contributory factor for a wide variety of emotional and mental health difficulties.

It can be comforting, as well as useful, to hear of other people's emotional and mental health experiences. But communicating how our brain is working and what we are feeling can be difficult, particularly as we each tend to use words and language in subtly different ways. Therefore some of the 'symptoms' below have been listed more than once because they have been described in more than one way.

It should not be forgotten that any of these potentially food-related 'moods' can arise from a combination of different influences and not solely due to the effects of food. And sometimes there won't be any obvious links between mood and food at all. Yet it is becoming more apparent how food can be a crucial contributory factor for a wide variety of emotional and mental health difficulties for many people.

Some Food–Mood Symptoms

addictions	fears	mood swings
aggression	feeling 'unreal'	nervousness
anxiety	forgetfulness	over-sensitive
apathy	hearing your own	painfully shy
autism	thoughts	panic attacks
behavioural disorders	high interest in sex	paranoia
can't think straight	hyperactivity	phobias
compulsions	ideas of grandeur	pre menstrual syndrome (PMS)
concentration difficulties	indifference	restlessness
cravings	illusions	rituals
crying	insomnia	seasonal affective
day-dreaming	irritability	disorder (SAD)
delinquency	lack of energy	seeing or hearing things
delusions	lack of sex drive	abnormally
depression	learning disabilities	schizophrenia
difficulty sleeping	light sleeper	sleep disorders
driven feeling	low interest in sex	spacey feeling
dyslexia	memory difficulties	suicidal thoughts
eating disorders	mental confusion	suspicious of people
emotional ups and downs	mental exhaustion	tension
fatigue	mood changes	tired all the time

Case Study: 'Brain Fatigue'

The summer before I became ill I began a strenuous new job. I also developed a keen sweet tooth, started to drink more tea than normal and often ate two large evening meals. I took a holiday to recharge my batteries but afterwards I found I couldn't get up in the mornings or get back into 'the swing of things' at work. I started making excuses for coming in late and going home early. (Previously I would work a 10–12-hour day and go to the gym on two or three days each week.) After two weeks of being desperately tired, always thirsty and generally low, I went to the doctor. I found myself crying about how tired I was and was ordered to 'sleep it off' for a few days. Yes, I slept, but I found I was even more tired after sleeping. I felt I had been running a marathon while I was asleep!

Going back to see the doctor, I had to persuade him I wasn't depressed and that I didn't need antidepressants. 'Signed off' from work by now, I was expecting to be back at work after just one or two weeks more. But instead I got worse and barely had the energy or inclination to get out of bed. Living on my own, my only motivation to get up was to make myself a cup of tea or a meal of pasta and chocolate! If I tried to get up and dressed in the hope of making myself feel better, I found that just the effort of pulling on a jogging suit exhausted me! Even my brain seemed to be tired.

This nightmare lasted over three months with fortnightly visits to the doctor who could only shrug his shoulders and say 'Hmm … this must be chronic fatigue syndrome but I know nothing about it except that you could be like this for two or more years.' At 29 and single, I was under threat of losing my job, my house and my social life. I was in a bad way.

Fortunately, my mum read an article about a nutritional therapist and I made an appointment. What a relief to find someone who could talk with me about how I felt. Most refreshing of all was being able to discuss the possible causes rather than just ways of treating the symptoms. After the first visit I stopped drinking caffeine and eating sugar and started on some vitamins. Within two weeks I saw my energy levels and my mental clarity begin to return. I could now bear to listen to the radio, watch TV and, more importantly, manage a few hours at work each day.

What became apparent as I started to feel better was how this illness had been affecting my brain. I have now gone back to working full time and I've got my life back. Although my memory isn't quite at its best, I do feel well and enjoy life. I now really understand the truth of the saying 'you are what you eat'! Even when I can relax a few elements of my diet I will never go back to the habits I had before.

Explanations

There are a number of different explanations for the cause-and-effect relationship between food and mood, and different foods can affect the body in different ways. The following are some examples:

- Brain chemicals influence the way we think, feel and behave (neurotransmitters such as serotonin, dopamine and acetylcholine). They can be affected by what's been eaten *(see Chapter 3)*.

- There can be abnormal reactions to artificial chemicals in foods, such as artificial colourings and flavourings, or to naturally-occurring chemicals in food such as the salicylates that are particularly high in certain fruits.

- There are reactions which can be due to the deficiency of an enzyme needed to digest a food. Lactase, for instance, is needed to digest lactose (milk sugar). Without it, a milk intolerance can build up.

- People can become hypersensitive to foods in a way that involves part of the immune system. This can result in so-called 'delayed' or 'hidden' food 'allergies' or 'sensitivities'.

- Low levels of vitamins, minerals and essential fatty acids can affect mental health, with some symptoms associated with particular nutritional deficiencies. For example, links have been demonstrated between low levels of certain B-vitamins and symptoms of schizophrenia, and low levels of the mineral zinc and eating disorders.

- High levels of certain toxins in the environment, such as lead from an excess of traffic pollution or mercury from leaky amalgam fillings, or vaccines, can also affect the proper functioning of the body and brain.

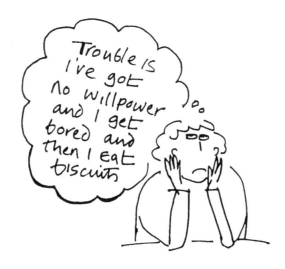

Pumpernickel with Tahini and Chopped Dates

Type:	Breakfast/Snack
Equipment:	Grill/Broiler
Preparation time:	1 min
Cooking time:	3 mins

Pumpernickel is a particular type of rye bread that can be purchased in packets of rectangular, flat slices. Other types of wholegrain rye bread are also suitable. These breads are ideal for those who need to avoid wheat and they are delicious toasted. Yeast-free versions are also available so check the labels. Pumpernickel and whole-grain rye breads have a low Glycaemic Index which means they release their energy slowly and so keep you going for longer. Tahini is sesame seed 'butter' which is higher in beneficial unsaturated fat than saturated fat. Tahini may be bought as 'light' or 'dark', depending on whether the seeds are hulled or not. Most of the good mood nutrients, including tryptophan protein, are contained in this breakfast or snack.

Ingredients (per person)

2–3 slices pumpernickel or whole-grain rye bread
1 tbsp dark or light tahini (sesame seed butter)
3 dried dates (chopped into small pieces)

Method

1   Spread the bread with tahini (margarine or butter is optional) and sprinkle with chopped dates.
2   Place under grill/broiler for approx. 3 mins.

Ready?	
Underdone	Not warmed through.
Just right	Beginning to 'sizzle' a little.
Overdone	Bread is burning and curling up at edges.

Trouble-shooting tip	This recipe is so easy it can't possibly go wrong!

Evidence

The scientific evidence that demonstrates the link between diet, nutrition and mental and emotional health is growing. However, it can be difficult to measure using the scientific method of the 'randomized, double-blind, placebo controlled trial'. This is where, for example, volunteers take capsules containing either an unknown food or 'dummy' capsules to test their reaction. Results can prove inconclusive when, for example, capsules do not contain enough food to cause a reaction, or if testing food sensitivities that are triggered through a combination of sight, smell and taste. Regrettably, problems such as these mean that medical practitioners who depend solely on scientific evidence can remain unconvinced that there is any association between food and mood.

This is unfortunate because there is plenty of other evidence for the food–mood connection, such as the positive responses from individuals who have made changes to their diets. These people can provide convincing, first-hand reports of the importance of certain foods for maintaining or improving their mental health and wellbeing. Also, there are the nutritional therapists who support individuals by guiding the process of making dietary changes and recommending appropriate nutritional supplementation. They are able to offer clinical evidence that food does affect mood.

People can provide convincing, first-hand reports of the importance of certain foods for maintaining or improving their mental health and wellbeing.

Common Culprits

The precise cause-and-effect relationship between different foods and moods has yet to be scientifically established, although individuals often find that they can associate certain foods with moods. The foods most commonly linked with mental and emotional symptoms are:

artificial additives (e.g. colourings such as tartrazine (E102), flavourings such as monosodium glutamate (MSG or E621), preservatives such as benzoic acid (E210)

chocolate
coffee
corn
eggs
milk and milk products (e.g. cheese, yoghurt, butter)
oranges

soya
sugar
tomatoes
wheat (e.g. bread, pasta, cakes, biscuits made from wheat flour)
yeast

It is important to remember that not all of these foods will be problem foods for most people – which is just as well, because this list probably describes many people's daily diets!

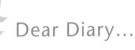

Dear Diary...

A diary can give you greater awareness of what you are doing and is an important first step towards making the appropriate alterations to your diet.

The recommended way to start the process of exploration into food and mood is to keep a diary of what you eat and drink and also how you feel. A diary can give you greater awareness of what you are doing and is an important first step towards making the appropriate alterations to your diet. Keeping a diary will give you an idea of what could be changed and, later on, will allow you to look back and see the effect of any changes you do make.

At first, the idea of writing everything down may seem something of a chore. Hopefully, after a while, you will be able to enjoy the process of reflecting on what you are doing and how you are feeling.

Some people choose to keep a diary as a way of controlling their diet. They have found that the discipline of writing down what they eat and drink helps them to change their eating habits. This can be especially powerful if you know you are going to share the contents of your diary with someone else. At the moment, however, we are considering diary-keeping as a method for finding out more information, rather than as a tool for changing behaviour.

Some benefits of keeping a food and mood diary:

- To record exactly what you are eating and drinking. People are often surprised when they look back over what they have eaten and discover that it is not quite what they thought it was!
- To enable you to draw up a list of 'prime suspects' for your investigation into food and mood.
- To discover any patterns in your eating and drinking that may be affecting how you feel, or which may be influencing your mental functioning.
- To enable you to monitor the effect of any changes you decide to make. The effects of making changes are often quite obvious and can result in dramatic improvements to health. However, if the benefits are less clear you will be able to look back to how things used to be and see what you've been able to achieve.

So, first let us consider how you could keep a diary. Then we'll look at what it can reveal about the relationship between the food you eat and the way you feel.

How to Keep a Food and Mood Diary

1   Find yourself a convenient-sized notebook that you can carry around with you. It seems to work best if you write down what you eat and drink at the time you have it. If you leave this to do at the end of the day you may find you have difficulty remembering accurately what you ate or drank.

2   Decide what information you would like to collect. The more information you include in your diary, the more useful it is likely to be. An example diary that shows the most important information you will need is given below. You may also like to include extra information – such as where you were and the approximate amounts you ate or drank.

3   Prepare the layout of the pages of your notebook according to the information you have decided to collect. Allow plenty of space and room for crossings out and extra notes. Refer to the sample page from below for an idea on the layout you might choose.

4   Make sure the diary is clearly marked as belonging to you, just in case you leave it somewhere by mistake. Mark it private if that is how you want to keep it. Clip a pen to the diary so there are no excuses for you not recording what you've just eaten!

5   Be prepared to redesign the content and layout of the pages as you learn what works for you. Keep the diary for at least one week. If you can maintain it for longer – say up to one month – then so much the better.

What Your Food and Mood Diary Could Reveal

It is often a combination of eating too much of some foods and not enough of others which can contribute to symptoms such as depression or anxiety.

Once you have kept your diary for at least one week, you can look back over the pages to find out more about what you are eating and how you are feeling. By looking at your diary and considering the following questions you will be able to draw up a list of suspect foods. This list of suspects is essential for the investigation process that follows in the next chapter. For each question that follows, you will be guided to the places in this handbook where you will be able to find further information on that topic.

Food and Mood Diary

Time & Date	What I eat/drink	How I feel physically	How I feel emotionally
Mon 12th			
8am	coffee (black, 2 sugars)	tired and aching (8)	irritable (6)
8.30am			irritable (1)
10am	doughnut	ditto	anxious (3)
11am	coffee (black, 2 sugars)	okay	anxious (5)
11.30am			'buzzy' (6)

Fig 12 – Food and Mood Diary

A Food and Mood Diary works best if it is kept in a clear and methodical manner. The more information the diary contains, the more useful it is likely to be. One suggestion for its layout is given above, together with an example of what the diary could contain.

It can be helpful to separate out the more physical and the more emotional symptoms.

Examples of physical symptoms you could record include: tired, headache, stomach ache, muscle aches, weakness. Examples of emotional or mental symptoms may include: feeling anxious, impulsive, restless, can't concentrate, forgetful, insomnia, irritable, restless, angry, depressed, shaky, bored, tearful. You may, of course, choose to include only the emotional or mental states that are strongest or of most concern to you, rather than documenting every subtle change in mood you might experience.

Rating symptoms provides you with a way of comparing symptoms and how you feel from one day to the next. One method is to give each symptom a score by rating it on a scale of 1 to 10, where 10 is the worst possible experience and 1 is very mild.

1. HOW MUCH ARE YOU EATING?

As far as food affecting mood is concerned, it is often a combination of eating too much of some foods and not enough of others which can contribute to symptoms such as depression or anxiety. So, a fundamental thing for you to consider will be: is there any one food, or type of food, that is being eaten every day (or nearly every day) or in particularly large amounts?

This is because the basis of a healthy diet is about achieving a balance between a wide variety of foods, where the variety – instead of being crammed into one day – is spread out over a number of days. Some foods – perhaps because they are generally considered healthy to eat – can be eaten on a daily basis by many people. Unfortunately, these can be the very foods that are having a disguised yet disabling influence upon your health.

You can use the contents of your Food and Mood Diary to complete the following exercise. This will help you to think about how often you eat the common culprit foods most often linked with emotional, mental and behavioural symptoms.

How Often Do You Eat These Foods?

How often do you eat (or drink) the following? For each food, tick the column that applies.

Food	More than twice a week	Less than twice a week
wheat products (e.g. bread, pasta, pastry, cakes)		
animal milk products (e.g. milk, cheese, yoghurt, butter, ice cream)		
yeast and foods containing yeast (e.g. yeast extract, bread, beer, wine, cheese, mushrooms)		
citrus fruit (i.e. oranges, lemons, limes, grapefruit)		
egg and foods containing egg (e.g. cakes, custard, quiche, meringue, batter, mayonnaise, ice cream)		
soya (e.g. soya milk, soya yoghurt, tofu, vegetarian sausages/ burgers)		
nightshade family (i.e. tomatoes, potatoes, aubergines, peppers, chillies, paprika)		
corn (e.g. sweetcorn, cornflakes, popcorn, corn oil, corn syrup)		

The foods that you eat on more than two occasions each week are the foods that need to go on your list of suspects.

2. WHAT TYPES OF FOOD DO I USUALLY EAT?

There are a number of ways of looking at the type of food you are eating. For example, starchy and sugary foods, foods that contain mostly fat or protein, foods that are a good sources of fibre, stimulant foods such as tea and coffee, and foods containing additives can all have different effects on mood. Have a look in your diary at what you usually eat and then consider the following:

1   Which, and how many, sweet or sugary foods do I eat each day?
2   Which, and how many, starchy carbohydrate foods (bread/pasta/potatoes) do I eat each day?
3   Which, and how many, protein foods (meat, fish, eggs, cheese, beans) do I eat each day?
4   Which, and how many, fibre-containing foods (vegetables, beans, wholegrains such as wholemeal bread, pasta or brown rice) do I eat each day?
5   Which, and how many, fat or oil-containing foods do I eat each day?
6   Which, and how many, alcoholic drinks, cups of coffee, tea, hot chocolate or cans of cola do I drink each day?
7   Which, and how many, foods containing additives (colourings, flavourings, preservatives) do I consume each day?

The importance for your emotional and mental health of these questions are explained in the following chapters of this handbook:

- What you eat can influence the levels of brain chemicals affecting your thinking, feeling, performance and behaviour. More information on this aspect of food is provided in Chapter 3.
- Diets and their effect on mood can be looked at in a number of ways and Chapter 2 introduced two Oriental systems of health care which recognize that foods can affect the mind.
- Foods can be grouped according to the botanical family they belong to. A sensitivity to one type of food may mean that close relatives of that food could also be having an effect. Chapter 6 contains details of food families and cross-reactions between close relatives.
- Foods and drinks such as coffee, tea, chocolate and cola contain caffeine which influence how we feel. More information on this subject can be found in Chapter 7.
- Blood sugar metabolism plays an important part in how we feel. Chapter 8 considers the foods that can influence – for better or worse – fluctuating blood sugar levels.
- Having enough good mood nutrients is essential for emotional and mental health. Make sure you are getting enough of what you need by reading Chapter 10.

3.WHAT ARE MY PATTERNS OF EATING?

For maintaining emotional and mental wellbeing, when you eat is as important as what you eat and how much. So, first, look back over your diary and consider the following:

1   Do I always eat breakfast?
2   Do I always eat lunch?
3   Do I always eat dinner?
4   Do I eat at (roughly) the same time each day?
5   Do I eat at set times or do I wait until I'm feeling hungry?
6   Do I eat and drink between meal times?

The significance of your answers to these questions is particularly important for keeping your blood sugar levels steady and your mood and energy on an even keel. More information on this important aspect of food and mood can be found in Chapter 8.

The effects of artificial additives on mood are often particularly obvious in children.

Some Links to Look Out for

By comparing what you eat and how you feel you may notice some links between food and mood. Here are some signs that can provide important clues:

1   If you feel noticeably better or obviously worse within an hour of eating or drinking something then that should arouse your suspicions. Instant benefits from eating a food can indicate an addictive-type relationship. This can occur with a number of different foods. For example, some people have headaches or feel that they cannot concentrate on what they are doing, then have a cup of coffee and feel much better very quickly. What could be happening here is that by drinking coffee you are 'topping up' to the level of caffeine your body needs to avoid experiencing the symptoms of caffeine withdrawal. (More information on the effects of coffee can be found in Chapter 7.)

2   Another, somewhat clearer, relationship between a food and mood can be seen in the effect of artificial additives such as colourings, flavourings and preservatives. The effects of these chemicals, which can include headaches, poor concentration or behavioural changes such as hyperactivity, can occur soon after eating or drinking the suspect foods. They are often particularly obvious in children. A list of potentially problematic additives is given in Chapter 6.

3   Starchy or sugary foods are other examples of foods that can make a more obvious difference to the way you feel. Here, there is likely to be a pattern of feeling better within an hour of eating which is followed by a 'dip' in mood and energy some hours later. The negative effect may be avoided by eating or drinking again before the dip occurs but, depending on what is eaten, this can set up another cycle of high followed by low. Relying on regular intakes of stimulating foods or drinks to avoid the rebound lows creates high levels of stress for the mind and body. More information on the effect of starch or sugary foods on mood can be found in Chapter 8.

4   It is likely that there will be more than one food that is having a detrimental effect on your emotional and mental health. Until you unravel the different relationships, the effect of any one food on how you feel is likely to be mixed up with the effects of other foods. This is known as 'masking' and is explained further in the next chapter. So, keep an open mind as you draw up your list of suspects.

Drawing Up Your List of Suspects

By looking over your Food and Mood Diary and thinking about what you are eating you should be able to compile a list of suspect foods that could be affecting your moods. You may already have had some suspicions as to the foods that may be 'disagreeing' with you in some way. So your list of suspects will probably comprise:

♣   Foods that you eat daily or several times a week.
     Foods which you like the most, may crave or even binge on. The foods we crave are often the foods we are in an addictive relationship with, and which can be undermining our health. Feeling worse if you don't eat a food or unpleasant symptoms that disappear when you do eat a food can be important clues to look for. A feeling of strong attachment to a food can also point to these suspects.

♣   Foods that you suspect 'disagree' with you in some way although you may not be clear exactly how.

♣   Foods on the list of common culprits. If you find you become stuck drawing up your suspects list, you may like to consider including one or more of the most common problem foods that have been linked with emotional and mental difficulties, provided earlier in this chapter.

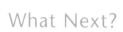

What Next?

So, you have kept a Food and Mood Diary for at least one week, collected observations about how you feel and noted what you ate and drank. You then carefully sifted through this valuable evidence for clues and searched for suspect foods that might be behind some of your symptoms. These prime suspects are now waiting to be investigated. Let's now find out if they are guilty.

'I began by keeping a diary of everything – yes everything – that I ate each day. This was quite revealing. I kept this up for a total of six weeks and this proved to be a straightforward system for monitoring my eating habits. The most useful and at times alarming part was putting a highlighter pen through the items that I needed to avoid or cut down on. And the more marker pen I used ...'

'I learned that it does matter what I eat and it's OK to look at food in a detailed way as it *will* affect me.'

'I was surprised at how little I ate and particularly how many cups of coffee I get through in just one day.'

Food and Mood Project participants

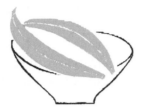

5

Investigations

Now that you have some idea which foods could be linked to how you are feeling, it's time to investigate their effects on your health so that you can be certain. Different foods affect the body in different ways and this handbook is concerned with foods and their effects on emotional and mental functioning.

The term 'allergy' was originally used to mean any type of 'altered reactivity' to a food. It is now often used to describe a very specific type of physical response involving the immune system. This handbook uses the term 'food sensitivity' to refer to any type of abnormal response to eating a food. In this chapter are guidelines for how you can investigate food sensitivities using a tried-and-tested, medically-approved method.

It can be helpful at this stage of your exploration into food and mood to consider any changes to your diet as being only short-term. Rather like a scientific experiment, the purpose of any alterations you make now will be simply to find out information. In other words, these changes are just a tool for revealing the effects of food on your moods. It is only once you have collected this information that you will be able to decide if longer-term changes to your diet are what's needed.

The elimination and challenge procedure described in this chapter is recognized as the 'gold standard' method for investigating food sensitivities. Even though you may not want to be too formal about conducting your investigations, you will find that the more methodical you are, the clearer will be the food and mood connections that you make.

Taking Care

If you want to be rigorous in carrying out your investigations, you will need to choose to make changes to what you eat at a time when there aren't other things happening in your life. Other things happening, or 'variables' (as scientists call them), could include events that affect the way you feel or occasions when you will already be eating new and different foods. Anniversary celebrations, birthdays, Christmas, holidays or stressful times at work are all familiar examples. When scientists design experiments they try and make sure that only one thing is going on at a time. In your experimentation with food and mood, careful planning to avoid confusion will make it clearer as to exactly what is having an effect on how you feel.

There are necessarily some costs associated with making changes, but these are usually rewarded by significant benefits to emotional and mental health.

It isn't just for the sake of clarity that the timing of a change in diet needs to be carefully thought about. Time and effort is involved in changing what you eat. As you try out new and different foods, for instance, you may find that you have to shop at unfamiliar places to obtain what you need. Smaller and slower changes introduced one at a time can be easier to manage. It is also easier to sustain gentle changes to your lifestyle, should you find them beneficial. Hopefully, you will enjoy the process of change and find it a positive experience. There are necessarily some costs associated with making changes, but these are usually rewarded by significant benefits to emotional and mental health.

Cutting Out or Cutting Down?

The disadvantage of 'cutting down' compared to 'cutting out' a suspect food is that cutting down may not produce such clear-cut results.

One way to investigate the effect of a suspect food on your emotional and mental health is simply to reduce the amount you consume and see if you notice a difference in how you feel. For example, consulting your Food and Mood Diary may reveal that you eat a lot of eggs. You discover that you have eggs in some shape or form on most days – perhaps boiled, scrambled, poached or fried or hidden in a cake. You consider them to be a convenient and nutritious food but they are now on your list of suspects and you want to find out if they are having any effect on your health.

ROTATION DIETS

If you choose to investigate the effect of eggs by cutting down, then you may still have some egg every day, but not as much as you usually do. Better still, you could have eggs on some days and not others. This approach is known as a rotation diet and will be looked at in more detail later on. But for now, the easiest type of rotation diet to describe is one known as a 'two day rotation'. To use this diet, you need to plan your meals so that you eat the suspect food – in this example it is eggs – only on alternate days. It is quite easy to stick to a two-day rotation diet if you follow the guideline of:

if I eat (eggs) today I won't eat them tomorrow
or (to put it another way)
if I ate (eggs) yesterday, I won't eat them today

ELIMINATION DIETS

The most thorough method of investigating suspect foods is when you 'cut out' a food from your diet completely. This is known as an 'elimination diet'. To use this approach (again taking eggs as an example), you would first note every possible source of eggs in your diet and then cut out eggs completely for a time.

Whilst you did this you would eat something else that was similar in the nutrition it provided but which didn't contain egg. (The next chapter provides some useful information on the hidden sources of suspect foods in your diet, along with nutritionally similar alternatives that you can substitute.) During this 'elimination diet', which usually takes from one to three weeks, you would pay close attention to how you were feeling to see if the change you had made was producing any results.

The disadvantage of 'cutting down' compared to 'cutting out' a suspect food is that cutting down may not produce such clear-cut results. The advantage is that it can be much easier to do, is less of a sudden change and less likely to produce withdrawal effects (see later section in this chapter). Some people like to cut down in stages before they finally cut out something completely. You will need to decide which is the best method to suit your personality and your lifestyle.

One Food or More?

Another decision you will need to make before you start your investigations is how many foods to test at any one time. Some people like to cut out all possible suspect foods in one go; others prefer to 'chip away' at the changes they want to make and cut out just one food at a time. Again, there are advantages and disadvantages to both approaches and you will need to decide which is likely to work best for you.

Tackling all the suspects at once is most likely to provide benefits in the shortest amount of time. It may also reduce the problem of masking *(see below)*. However, removing all suspects in one go is likely to produce more withdrawal symptoms and create the most inconvenience for you. Then, because you won't know which of the foods on your list of suspects are the problem (or culprit) foods, you will need to do a further investigation in order to find out. This next step is usually known as a 'challenge' and is explained below.

The alternative to cutting out all suspects at once is 'chipping away'. Chipping away by changing one food at a time is easier to manage practically and it can reduce withdrawal symptoms. But as a method of revealing culprit foods, its big disadvantage is that it can take much longer. It can also be inconclusive because of the 'masking' effect of foods.

Comparison Between Cutting Out and Cutting Down

All suspects at once	One suspect at a time
1. Produces greatest benefits in the shortest amount of time.	1. Can take longer to get any obvious benefit.
2. Can avoid the problem of food effects masking each other.	2. Can be inconclusive if the effect of one food is masking the effect of another.
3. More withdrawal symptoms likely.	3. Fewer withdrawal symptoms likely.
4. More inconvenience, more stress.	4. Less inconvenience, less stress.
5. A one-by-one 'challenge' of each food is then needed to confirm the effect of eating each individual food.	5. A food 'challenge' may be needed to confirm the effect of eating the food.

Masking

It is quite easy for some reactions to be attributed to the wrong food.

Rather like an addiction, a food you are sensitive to can create feelings of 'stimulation' before the more obviously negative effects start to take hold. The negative effects of a food may become apparent as your body starts to crave another 'hit' of the food. If this is not soon satisfied the result can be unpleasant withdrawal symptoms.

To complicate matters, you are more likely to be sensitive to several foods than to just one. This means that the obvious effect of any one food on your mood can be masked by the effect of another food. Any cause-and-effect relationship between a food and the symptoms it provokes can be tangled up with the cause-and-effect relationship of another food and its symptoms. It is therefore quite easy for some reactions to be attributed to the wrong food. Alternatively, some reactions may go unnoticed altogether – because they have been 'upstaged' by the effect of another food. And the more problem foods you are eating regularly, the greater is this masking effect.

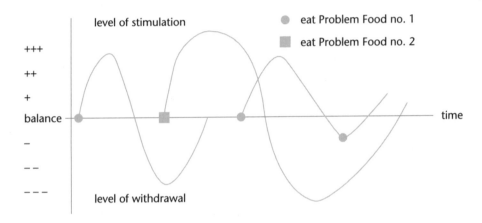

Fig 13 – Masking

Problem Food no. 1 (●) produces stimulatory effects. If another 'dose' of the food isn't taken, withdrawal symptoms are experienced which eventually diminish as balance is regained. Eating more of the same food negates the withdrawal process. (This cycle can feel similar to the roller-coaster ride produced by fluctuating blood sugar levels described in Chapter 8.)

As the stimulatory effects of Problem Food no. 1 diminish and withdrawal symptoms begin, another food, Problem Food no. 2 (■), may be eaten. The effect on the body of eating Problem Food no. 2 produces a similar cycle of highs and lows.

The low produced by the withdrawal effect of avoiding Food no. 1 is now masked by the stimulatory effect of Food no. 2.

The more problem foods that are eaten, the more complete is the masking of the related symptoms. This can make it impossible to know which food is associated with which effect. It is only as successive foods are removed from the diet that the underlying fluctuations in health related to diet become apparent.

You may be wondering why the masking effect of culprit foods is considered a problem, particularly when the negative withdrawal effects of one food appear to be counterbalanced by the stimulatory effect of another food. This masking is cause for concern as it represents a condition of stress for the body. And prolonged stress eventually takes its toll on health. It can be thought of as the state of imbalance which was described in Chapter 1 as the 'adaptation stage' of the General Adaptation Syndrome. Sustained adaptation to negative effects of food depletes the body of resources and cannot last for long.

Keeping Records

A well-kept diary can help you to be more objective about how you feel.

Whilst you conduct your investigation it is particularly important to keep a record of how you feel. A daily diary of changes to symptoms will enable you to compare more accurately how you are feeling now with how you felt days or weeks earlier. It is very easy to forget how you felt and imagine that things were either worse (or better) than they actually were. A well-kept diary can help you to be more objective about how you feel.

This next diary is somewhat different to the Food and Mood Diary which you used to draw up your list of suspects. A sample layout, with an example of the information it could contain, is given below.

- This Diary will be kept for a period of one to three weeks. As you will probably only be able to fit a few days on each page, you will need to redraw the diary grid every few days.
- For each page of the diary, draw two columns, one where you can list the symptoms you wish to monitor, the other (which will be wider) where you can grade the severity of those symptoms on each successive day.
- Then, further divide the second column into one column labelled 'before' followed by a separate column for each new day.

SYMPTOMS	SEVERITY (0 = symptom free, 10 = worst possible)					
	BEFORE	DAY 1	DAY 2	DAY 3	DAY 4	DAY 5
irritable	(3–7)	6–8	6–7	3–5	1–2	0
depressed	7	9	8	7	6	5

Fig 14 – Withdrawal Diary

1   Before beginning the changes to your diet, complete the first column of the Withdrawal Diary which asks you to list the symptoms you wish to monitor during the withdrawal period. Include any aspect of your health you are concerned about, whether or not you think it is related to what you are eating or drinking.

2   Grade the symptoms in the 'before' column according to how you have experienced them

during the last few weeks. Put a 10 for the worst possible and reserve 0 for a symptom that disappears completely. You can give a single score to represent the worst a symptom gets during the day or choose a 'rough average' score for the day. Either is fine, just make sure you stick with one system or the other. If symptoms vary throughout the day you may prefer to give a score that is a range of two numbers – the higher number being the worst you feel and the lower number being the best you feel in any one day. An example of a scoring system that uses a single number and one that uses a range is shown in the diary example above.

3   When you decide to make the change to your diet that involves cutting out a culprit food, you will start a withdrawal period and experience a change in how you feel. So, for each day that follows, give a score for each of the symptoms you have listed in the first column. If any new symptoms appear, list them in the first column and give them a score under the appropriate day. Continue monitoring how you feel on a daily basis for up to three weeks.

Withdrawal

Withdrawal symptoms are simply the body readjusting to the change in diet and they will improve within a few days. You can see them as a sign that you are on the right track and feel encouraged.

If the food(s) you have chosen to investigate is the food guilty of causing you some symptoms then, when you remove it from your diet (or reduce the amount you eat), you are likely to experience some withdrawal symptoms. This can be a worsening of how you usually feel and may include symptoms that you haven't experienced for a while or even some that are completely new to you.

Withdrawal symptoms are simply the body readjusting to the change in diet and they will improve within a few days. You can see them as a sign that you are on the right track and feel encouraged. Your Withdrawal Diary can help track this process for you and make it clearer. In your diary you will probably begin by recording a worsening of symptoms (where your scores get higher) for the first few days, after which you start to feel much better and the scores will start to go down.

Withdrawal symptoms should improve after about one week. If they continue beyond this time then they could be due to something other than the change to your diet and you should consult your doctor. In fact, any symptoms you are concerned about at any time following a change to your diet should be discussed with your doctor. Explain what you have been doing and hopefully you will be reassured that you will be feeling much better soon.

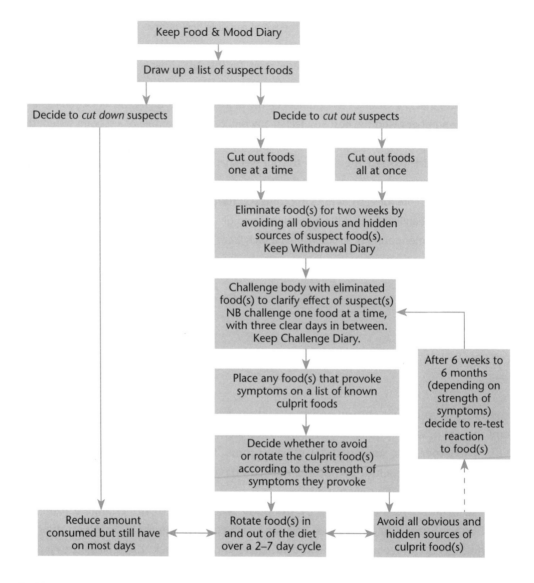

Fig 15 – Food Sensitivity Investigations

Unclear Results

Often, efforts to change what you eat will be rewarded with an obvious improvement in how you feel and there is a clear link between foods and moods. But there are occasions when this relationship isn't quite as convincing. In these cases, you will have altered your diet by cutting out a food but, despite keeping a careful record of the changes in your health that followed, you are still unsure if you've found the culprit food.

Another scenario is that you decided to cut out several foods all at once. Your health has noticeably improved and you are feeling much better, but the new diet is proving difficult to keep going and you don't want to be avoiding a food unnecessarily. You need to know exactly which of the foods you have cut out are the culprit foods, guilty of making you feel worse should you eat them.

Both these scenarios can be successfully addressed by doing an experiment, one that is usually called a 'challenge'. This experiment is called a challenge because the same food (or foods) that you cut out is used to 'challenge' the body, to see if any symptoms are provoked through eating it. You can then assume that if you feel worse after reintroducing a food that you had been avoiding, the deterioration in your health is due to the effect of the food.

Doing a 'Challenge'

When you reintroduce a food to see if it makes you feel worse, the clearest results are obtained in the following way:

- if you eat the food first thing in the morning on an empty stomach (should you eat something in the evening, it is possible that any symptoms produced will occur at night and are then missed because you are asleep)
- if you eat a substantial portion of the food
- if you eat the food by itself or with foods you are certain you are not sensitive to
- if you eat the food without the addition of spices, condiments, sugar etc. which could confuse the results.

Again, doing the challenge experiment in a methodical way will yield the clearest information for you. Therefore, keeping a Challenge Diary can be very helpful.

This diary records the time you eat a food and what you eat, and then provides space for you to record the time and severity of any symptoms that may follow.

Date	Time	Food/drink	Time	Symptom	Severity (0–10)
3rd April	8.15am	bread	8.45am	fuzzy head	8
			9.45am	very tired	9
				depressed	7

Fig 16 – Challenge Diary

Positive Results

When you do a 'challenge', you will have increased any sensitivity you may have to the food in question because you have been avoiding it for about two weeks. This is rather like the 'recovery stage' of the General Adaptation Syndrome (*see Chapter 1*), where avoidance of a problem substance increases your sensitivity to it. This increased sensitivity makes it easier for you to spot any effects the food might have.

The symptoms that can be provoked by food are wide ranging. They can include an unexpected feeling of tiredness or an unexplained change in mood. They may last for a few hours or less but could continue until your body is completely clear of that food which, depending on your digestive system and metabolism, may take two to three days.

When you perform a food challenge you also need to be aware of two possible complications: late (or delayed) reactions and strong reactions.

LATE REACTIONS

The majority of symptoms appear within one to six hours after eating the food. However, some symptoms can take two to three days to appear after the food has been eaten.

So, if you don't get any symptoms on the first 'challenge', repeat it by eating the food again at the next meal. If after three challenges (i.e. one at breakfast, lunch and dinner that day) no symptoms are noticed, stop eating that food but continue to record your symptoms for the next three days. If, after three more days, there are no obvious effects from eating the food, you can assume that it is not a problem for you.

STRONG REACTIONS

At the challenge stage, any sensitivity you may have to the suspect food under investigation can be increased, so that when you reintroduce the food, symptoms are produced which – for some people – can be difficult to deal with. It is important to be aware of this possibility so that you are prepared to cope. If you are concerned about this possibility then it would be wise to explain to a family member or friend that you are investigating the effects of food. Tell them that you may feel unwell for a short time following the reintroduction of the food you have been avoiding, and check that they will be sympathetic.

Warning

People with some physical health conditions need to be aware that a food challenge can exacerbate their symptoms. For example, someone with asthma could feel wheezy for a while after challenging their body with a suspect food that they have been avoiding. A heart condition or high blood pressure could also be made temporarily worse. **It is very important that anyone with a potentially serious medical condition consult their doctor before doing a food elimination and challenge.**

Tip: Health Salts

A simple and often effective remedy that can be used to reduce an unpleasant reaction to food is to immediately take 1–2 level teaspoons of sodium bicarbonate in a glass of water. Sodium bicarbonate (sometimes called 'Health Salts') is available from any pharmacy.

Case Study: Depression

Teresa had several concerns about her physical and emotional health which included periodically feeling irritable, angry and depressed for no obvious reason. She agreed to try an elimination and challenge diet for the two most likely suspects which were wheat-containing foods (such as wheat-based bread and pasta) and cow's milk (including foods made from milk such as cheese, yoghurt and butter). During this time she cut out all obvious and hidden sources of these foods and kept a diary of her symptoms. When she looked back over the diary, it clearly showed the link between the changes she had made to her diet and how she was now feeling.

Teresa's emotional symptoms hadn't been her main concern but she had decided to record everything about how she felt – both physically and emotionally. As she began the elimination stage (of the elimination and challenge diet), Teresa initially felt worse as she started to withdraw from these frequently-eaten foods. Her diary showed how the score she had given to the symptoms of feeling angry and depressed had suddenly increased. Then, as time progressed, the score for these symptoms declined steadily to zero as Teresa began to feel better. It seemed that she was on the right track in choosing to cut out foods containing wheat and cow's milk, but to make certain these foods were connected to how she felt, Teresa then tried the 'challenge' stage.

It was important to challenge the body with only one of the two foods she had been eliminating at a time. If she was to eat bread and cheese together, for example, and then felt worse, it wouldn't be possible to say which food was the culprit. Teresa decided to start with cow's milk and the food she was going to use as the 'challenge food' was cheese. As it was a work day, Teresa ate early and had a good-sized portion of cheese with an apple. Although she was on the lookout for a physical reaction, she was surprised at the strength of the emotional impact that followed her breakfast. Mid-morning, Teresa recorded in her diary that she was feeling very emotional and weepy, giving this feeling a score of 7 out of a possible 10. She also felt extremely constipated. Teresa continued to eat cheese at every meal that day and later that evening was suffering with an upset stomach. The link between cheese and feeling ill was quite clear, but to be absolutely certain, Teresa repeated the experiment a few weeks later, with similarly unpleasant effects.

When Teresa tried the wheat challenge she experienced a delayed reaction for the emotional symptoms. The day after she had eaten some pasta, as well as feeling physically ill, Teresa felt very low, weepy and that she 'couldn't cope'.

Now convinced that both wheat- and milk-containing foods were off the menu for the time being, Teresa needed advice on what she could eat during a forthcoming walking holiday. She decided that a hearty cooked breakfast or a steaming bowl of oat porridge made with water would help her through the day. She would travel equipped with oatcakes or rice cakes to replace the bread in the (provided) packed lunches and take special care to avoid cheese sandwich fillings!

Testing More than One Food

If you have eliminated more than one food then the challenge experiment needs to be done for one food at a time so that you are clear about the results. And because of the possibility of late reactions, sufficient time has to be allowed between challenges before testing the next food. This is to ensure your body has had a chance to clear itself of the first food. Leaving three days between challenges is usually sufficient.

What to Do if You Get a Reaction

The good news is that if you do discover a culprit food which provokes an unpleasant reaction for you, then your body's response to it can be changed.

If a food does provoke a symptom you will have valuable information that will help you decide whether or not to continue eating that food. If you have a strong reaction, it is likely that you will want to avoid that food because you have clearly demonstrated its negative effect on your health. Less strong reactions may leave you feeling somewhat uncertain as to what to do for the best. This is where a compromise may be needed, and a rotation diet (*see Chapter 6*) can be the solution. One consideration is likely to be how easy it will be for you to obtain the alternative food(s) you would need to substitute for the culprit food. Some practical considerations related to a change in what you eat can be found in the next chapter.

Fortunately, the type of sensitivity to foods we are exploring are not necessarily life-long conditions. So, the good news is that if you do discover a culprit food which provokes an unpleasant reaction for you, then your body's response to it can be changed. What will be needed, however, is a period of avoiding the food which, according to your particular sensitivity, could be a few weeks or may be several months.

After this period of avoidance you will probably find that you can enjoy the food once more without experiencing unpleasant symptoms. To maintain the benefits of your new-found tolerance to the food, it will be wise to eat the food only 'every-so-often' rather than every day. This approach to preventing food sensitivities from recurring or becoming worse uses a 'rotation diet' and it is discussed more fully in the next chapter.

Some Other Clues

The method of cutting down or cutting out foods (and seeing how you feel) and then reintroducing the food (and again seeing how you feel) is a tried and tested way of diagnosing food-related symptoms. The self-observations you make during the 'elimination and challenge' process are all you will need to make a judgement on which foods are beneficial for you to eat and which are not. However, to confirm your subjective observations, you may also like to use what are considered to be more objective observations and measurements on how your body is affected by food. These are not, however, 100 per cent conclusive evidence, so they are best used only to back up your subjective observations.

One option is for you to enlist the help of a trusted friend who can notice how you appear to them as you change your diet. It can be particularly useful to hear someone else's opinion on how you are after you reintroduce a food you have been avoiding. Another person's view of how you seem needs to be considered along with your own subjective experience. Their observations are neither more (nor less) valid than your own.

Other more objective measurements which you can easily make at home involve changes to weight, pulse rate and body temperature. Of course, it is important to be aware that there may be other reasons for a change in weight, pulse rate or body temperature and these measurements cannot be used on their own to make a diagnosis of food sensitivity.

WEIGHT CHANGES

A daily fluctuation in body weight of about 1lb (approx. 0.5kg) is considered normal. Greater than this may be due to changes in the level of water retention in the body, caused by a negative reaction to food. The following are the steps you will need to take to use changes in body weight as a method of confirming a food sensitivity.

1   Before you make any changes to your diet, record your weight (unclothed and with an empty bladder). Do this first thing in the morning and last thing at night before you start the elimination diet. This is to see how your weight fluctuates before you change your diet.

2   Start the elimination diet. At the end of the two weeks' elimination, record your weight once more. Do this first thing in the morning and last thing at night (unclothed and with an empty bladder). Compare this weight with your weight before you started the elimination diet. Any change in weight at this stage is likely to be due to the change in your diet. This is because when you eliminate a suspect food that you have a sensitivity to, a loss of weight in the form of water (that was being retained by the body in response to eating that food) is often the welcome result. Some people can lose several pounds (or kilograms) in one week, just through the body being able to let go of stored water.

3   During the challenge phase of your investigations, each day that you challenge the body with a new food, record your weight (morning and evening) as previously. In this case, if you have eaten a food that disagrees with you, your weight is likely to increase as your body holds on to water once more. Any increase in weight in excess of 1lb (approx. 0.5kg) can be taken as confirmation of a sensitivity to the food you have used to challenge the body.

PULSE CHANGES

An increase in your pulse rate can also be used to confirm a negative reaction to a food. This method can be used when challenging the body with the suspect foods that have been previously eliminated. This method is described below.

1   Measure your pulse by feeling with the finger tips of one hand along the side of your arm, just below the wrist of the other hand. Count the number of times your heart beats for a full one minute. Do this only after you have been sitting down quietly for five

minutes and not whilst smoking, eating or drinking. Write down your heart rate per minute.

2   Eat a portion of the suspect food and measure your pulse again, as described above. Record your heart rate. Any increase in heart rate of more than approximately 10 beats per minute is indicative of a reaction to a food. This may be followed minutes or hours later with emotional, mental or physical symptoms.

3   If there is no change to your heart rate immediately after you have eaten the food, you can try repeating this procedure 20, 40 and 60 minutes after eating the challenge food. Pulse changes later in the day may also indicate a reaction to the food eaten previously but are not as conclusive.

TEMPERATURE CHANGES

Although this measurement is less widely used in association with testing for food sensitivity, a low body temperature or a decrease in body temperature may indicate that culprit foods have been eaten. If your basal temperature is low before you start an elimination diet, it could be associated with a sensitivity to a food you are eating. If it falls following a food challenge, then a reaction to the food being tested may be the explanation.

To measure your body temperature you can use the Barnes Basal Temperature Test which may also be used to test for an underactive thyroid. You will need to ascertain your usual body temperature before you make any changes to your diet so that you can compare it with readings you make during the withdrawal and after a food challenge.

1   Before you go to bed, put a thermometer by the bed, together with paper and pen.

2   The next morning before you get up (even just to go to the toilet), use the thermometer to take the temperature under your arm. Do this by clamping the bulb end of the thermometer in your armpit, holding it in place with your arm for about 10 minutes. Do not talk or move until the 10 minutes is up. Then read the thermometer and make a note of your temperature.

3   Repeat this the following morning, preferably the same time as before, and then also for a third day. This is to gain an average basal body temperature measurement. Women who have periods need to do this on the second, third and fourth days of their period. Men, pre-pubescent and post-menopausal women may choose any three consecutive days.

4   A body temperature measured in this way which falls within the range 97.8–98.2°F (or 36.6–36.8°C) is considered normal. A temperature less than this could be due to a food sensitivity and an associated thyroid-function-depressing effect.

Food Sensitivity Tests

It is wise to think carefully, and find out as much as you can about a test, before undertaking any privately-funded food-sensitivity testing.

As long as you conduct your inquiries in the methodical manner described, and keep a clear record of your results, you should be able to find out how foods affect your moods. Investigations that cut down or cut out suspect foods give you complete control and can be conducted at a pace and in a way that suits your lifestyle. Yet these personal investigations do take time and effort and you may wonder if there are any other options open to you.

There are a number of different food sensitivity tests available which provide an alternative to the elimination and challenge procedure already described. The tests that doctors use are often limited to testing for classical food allergies only. Tests for classical food allergies measure the immune system's response to a food and the amount of IgE antibodies that are produced. You may already know if you have this type of reaction to a food as it produces immediate and obvious symptoms that are unlikely to be missed. Classical food allergy can even be life-threatening and is often associated with foods such as peanuts or shellfish, although other foods can be involved.

The type of food sensitivity we are concerned with is different to this classical, IgE mediated, food allergy. The negative response your body can have to foods which results in emotional or mental symptoms does not usually show up with this type of testing for IgE antibodies. There are several reasons why you may react inappropriately to foods and many alternative testing methods are being developed and offered to the public. However, a lot of these alternative tests are dismissed by many medical practitioners, some of whom even question the existence of these hidden or delayed food sensitivities.

In the absence of a medically approved test, most of the alternative tests that are available have to be paid for privately. The prices charged between different types of test vary as much as the methods of testing that are used. It is therefore wise to think carefully, and find out as much as you can about a test, before undertaking any privately funded food-sensitivity testing.

If you do decide to go ahead with a food sensitivity test, do remember that your response to a food will change as soon as you start to make changes to your diet. This may explain why different tests taken by the same person at different times can produce different results. However, if taken before you make any changes to what you eat, tests can provide useful information to guide you. When taken after you have started changing your diet, they may confirm what you have already discovered for yourself.

Millet Porridge

Type:	Breakfast
Equipment:	Medium pan and hob
Preparation time:	30 seconds
Cooking time:	5 minutes

Millet is rarely a cause of food sensitivity and may even have antifungal properties of benefit to those with a yeast overgrowth in the gut. The dried apricots used in this recipe have a particularly low Glycaemic Index, are a good source of antioxidants and minerals and even contain some tryptophan protein. Buy the darker-colour, unsulphured dried apricots if at all possible in order to avoid the possibility of reactions to the preservative – they also taste sweeter!

Ingredients (per person)

85g/3oz/1 cup millet flakes
500ml/1 pint/2 cups water or milk of your choice
2–3 dried apricots

Method

1   Place millet and water or milk into pan.
2   Snip dried apricots with scissors into the pan.
3   Heat over a medium temperature, stirring for most of the time.

Ready?
Underdone	Can still see individual flakes.
Just right	Thick, creamy consistency.
Overdone	As above but starting to stick to the pan and burn.

Trouble-shooting tips	Porridge is a lump rather than a creamy texture because there is not enough liquid – add some more water or milk.
	Porridge too runny – simmer without pan lid to evaporate off some of the liquid.

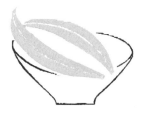

6

Sources and Substitutes

To investigate the effects of a suspect food on your mood you need to know when you are eating it! Much of the food we eat is ready-prepared or processed and can contain some surprising ingredients. This chapter provides information on where you may find the 10 most common culprit foods that could be linked with your symptoms. Whether you are cutting down, cutting out completely, or rotating a food in and out of your diet, you will need to be aware of the alternative foods you can substitute. So this chapter also provides some suggestions for tasty foods you can have instead.

 ## Getting Ready to Change Your Diet

It is a good idea to spend at least one week preparing for a change to your diet. This preparation time is when you continue having your usual food whilst you get used to being a 'food detective'. When shopping, cooking or eating you now need to get into the habit of noticing the ingredients of the meal or snack that you are having. If you find that it contains something you are wanting to eat less of, or to cut out completely, you will need to think about what you could have instead.

   If you are planning to be very thorough in your food-sensitivity investigations, you will also need to start reading food labels very carefully to check for hidden ingredients. This is important because, if during the process of elimination and challenge that follows, you have even a small amount of the food you are testing, it can confuse the results of your 'experiment'.

   During this 'getting ready' stage it is useful to make a note of the sources in your diet of the food(s) you are planning to change. Then you can list the alternatives you plan to substitute, which you will need to obtain before you can make any changes. An example of how you might go about this is given below.

1   For each food you are planning to investigate, use a new page in your notebook and divide it into two columns.

2   Label the first column 'sources' and the second column 'substitutes'.

3   Carry your notebook with you so that every time you eat something you can make a note of where the suspect food is hidden in your diet.

4   When your research is complete, use the second column to list the alternative foods that you will need to substitute instead. This column can then double up as a shopping list.

Food under investigation: e.g. wheat

Sources:	Substitutes:
Breakfast:	
Weetabix cereal	cornflakes
Lunch:	
cheese sandwich	rye crackers with cheese
Snack:	
biscuits	oat flapjack
Dinner:	
pasta and stir-fried vegetables	brown rice and stir-fried vegetables

Fig 17 – Getting Ready diary page

Being a Food Detective

It can help to develop a somewhat suspicious attitude to what you buy and eat.

To be an effective detective, you will need to get into the habit of reading food labels. The ingredients shown on packets and tins list foods in descending order of quantity. This means that something that is listed at the end will only be present in very small amounts and so possibly won't be worth worrying about. Constituents of a food that make up less than 25 per cent of the total product (the salami topping on a pizza, for example), and which may contain a mixture of foods, may not have their ingredients listed individually and may therefore require further investigation.

It can help to develop a somewhat suspicious attitude to what you buy and eat and remember that labels and ingredients lists can change. This extra-careful attitude to obtaining food won't be necessary every time you go shopping, but it is worth periodically rechecking labels of prepared foods you buy as their contents may change.

Another source of information are the food manufacturers themselves; their contact details can usually be found on the product label. Food stores have customer service departments which can usually provide lists of their own products suitable for those with special dietary needs. If you are eating out, many restaurants are now aware of the need to cater for special diets, and the waiting staff can be requested to ask the chef about the contents of a dish you would like to order.

Artificial Additives

Artificial additives can be found in most prepared and packaged foods such as tinned, packet, frozen and dried produce. Also in drinks in cans, cartons and bottles, particularly those that are artificially coloured and flavoured. Nutritional supplements and medicines can also contain additives. Toothpaste, cosmetics and toiletries are other potential sources of additives which can get into the body. Household cleaning products may be a problem and chemical sensitivity is an increasing concern for many food sensitive people.

Not all artificial additives are harmful to health and many additives are essential to preserve the freshness of processed and prepared foods. Unless you buy fresh foods and prepare all your meals from the basic ingredients, it is almost impossible to avoid artificial additives completely. However, by avoiding brightly coloured foods and drinks and checking labels you can avoid the worst offenders. Additives may be listed on food packaging by their full name or by the corresponding 'E-number'. They may also be referred to using vague terms such as 'colour' or 'flavour'. Some artificial additives to try and avoid, which include food colourings, flavourings and preservatives, have been listed below.

Additives to Avoid

Colourings

Allura Red AC	E129
Amaranth	E123
Brilliant Black BN	E151
Ponceau 4R, Conchineal Red A	E124
Sunset Yellow, FCF, Orange Yellow S	E110
Tartrazine	E102

Flavourings

Aspartame	E951
Monosodium glutamate (MSG)	E621
Saccharin, saccharin Na, K, Ca salts	E954

Preservatives

Benzoic acid	E210
Butylated hydroxy-anisole	E320
Calcium benzoate	E213
Calcium sulphite	E226
Potassium benzoate	E212
Potassium nitrate	E249
Propyl p-hydroxy-benzoate propyl-paraben, paraben	E216
Sodium metabisulphite	E223
Sodium sulphite	E221
Stannous chloride (tin)	E512
Sulphur dioxide	E220

The Top 10 Culprit Foods

The top 10 culprit foods most often found associated with emotional and mental-health difficulties are listed below in alphabetical order. For each food you will find:

- The main food sources of that food.
- The main drinks that could contain the culprit *(see also the table of common foods in alcoholic drinks later in this chapter)*.
- Other foods to watch out for, likely to have the culprit hidden among their ingredients.
- Close relatives of the food to help you continue your investigations if needed. Note that some people react to cooked versions of a food but not raw, and vice versa, so it is worth testing these as separate food items.
- Label reading tips.
- Related risks possible from non-food sources.
- Substitute and alternative foods and drinks you could have instead.

Sensitivity to caffeine and to sugar have been covered separately (in Chapters 7 and 8 respectively) and you may prefer to skip ahead and read these chapters first. How scrupulous you need to be in spotting every source of a suspect food in your diet will depend on how thorough you are wanting to be with your investigations. You may want to start by cutting down (or cutting out) just the main food and drink sources of a suspect or culprit, as it can be very hard to avoid some foods completely. A nutritional therapist can help by pointing out any food sources in your diet which you may have missed, and will also be able to provide guidance on maintaining a nutritionally balanced diet whilst you are avoiding certain foods.

> **Note:** if you have a classical, or IgE-mediated, food allergy and therefore need to be very careful about the contents of what you are eating, please be aware that the lists provided in this handbook cannot include every possible source of each culprit food and are intended as a guide only.

1. Chocolate

(See Chapter 2 for more information on chocolate cravings.)

Main food sources: biscuits, cakes, chocolate bars, desserts, sweets.

Main drink sources: chocolate milk shakes, cocoa drinks, 'hot' chocolate drinks.

Watch out for: chocolate as an ingredient or as a flavouring in other prepared and processed foods.

Close relatives: the caffeine in chocolate is also found in coffee, tea and cola *(see also Chapter 7)*. Chocolate contains a natural substance called phenylethylamine which is also found in red wine and cheese.

Label-reading tips: look for 'chocolate', 'cocoa' or 'caffeine'.

Related risks (non-food): none known.

Foods to have instead: the closest substitute for chocolate is carob. This is made from the carob bean and does not contain caffeine. It is available as confectionery and is used as a flavouring in some desserts and ice creams. It can also be purchased as a spread or as powder for baking or using in milk shakes or sauces. Other alternatives to chocolate that have a similar sweet and creamy nutty taste are nut butters. Almond, hazelnut and cashew nut butters are all high in beneficial polyunsaturated fats and are free from caffeine. These can be used in a variety of imaginative ways including as a spread, as a sauce and in milk shakes.

2. Coffee

(See Chapter 7 for more information on caffeine.)

Main food sources: coffee cake, coffee creams in chocolate assortments, coffee ice-cream.

Main drink sources: coffee drinks, including iced coffee.

Watch out for: coffee-flavouring in cakes, ice creams and other prepared and processed foods.

Close relatives: the caffeine in coffee is also found in tea, chocolate and cola. The herb guarana may also contain caffeine.

Label-reading tips: look for 'coffee', 'caffeine', 'cola nuts' or unidentified flavourings.

Related risks (non-food): none known.

Foods to have instead: there are many coffee substitutes and alternatives. *See Chapter 7 for several suggestions.*

3. Corn (Maize)

Main food sources: corn breakfast cereals, corn crisps, corn flour, corn 'niblets', corn oil, corn-on-the-cob, polenta, popcorn, sweet corn, taco shells, tortillas.

Main drink sources: ales, beers, lager, spirits, wine, glucose 'sports' drinks.

Watch out for: bakery goods, baking powder, custard, glucose powder, sweets and tablets, instant coffee, mixed grain breakfast cereals, nutritional supplements, sauces and gravy mixes, snacks, vegetable oil and many other prepared and processed foods.

Close relatives: other members of the grass family *(see 'Food Families' table later in this chapter).*

Label-reading tips: look for words containing, 'corn', 'dextrose', 'dextrin'. Words containing 'starch', 'maize', 'sweetening', 'syrup', 'vegetable' may refer to corn. Sugars such as fructose, glucose, sucrose, isomaltose and sorbitol can be derived from corn.

Related risks (non-food): adhesive gum on labels, stamps, envelopes (so spit rather than lick!). Tablets and medication (ask your pharmacist or doctor about obtaining medication in a form that does not use corn derivatives). Also starch on cotton clothes and starch used to seal and stiffen paper, card and cartons. Cosmetics and toiletries.

Foods to have instead: as for wheat (but excluding corn).

4. Eggs

Main food sources: batter, boiled eggs, omelette, poached eggs, quiche, scrambled eggs, scotch egg, soufflés.

Main drink sources: advocaat; egg may be used as a clarifier (fining) in soft drinks such as root beer or beer and wine.

Watch out for: bakery goods, custard, desserts, glazes on pastry, ice cream, lemon curd, mayonnaise, meringue, mousse, noodles, pancakes, pasta, pavlova, salad cream, sauces, Quorn, waffles, and many other prepared and processed foods.

Close relatives: chicken meat and other members of the pheasant family. Sometimes an apparent reaction to eggs is, in fact, a reaction to what the chicken has been fed (e.g. corn, soya, wheat)!

Label-reading tips: look out for words containing 'albumen', 'egg', 'globulin', 'livetin', 'ovalbumin', 'ovoglobulin', 'ovomucin', 'ovomucoid', 'ovovitellin', 'Simplesse', 'vitellin'. 'Emulsifier' 'lecithin' 'E322' may be derived from egg.

Related risks (non-food): egg shampoo, photographic film, some fabrics, some vaccinations.

Foods to have instead: egg 'replacers' for baking are available from health-food shops and mail-order suppliers. Duck and quail eggs may be suitable but as they are in the same food family they should be tested individually. Otherwise choose to eat another food from the meat, fish and vegetarian alternatives food group *(see Chapters 2 and 11).*

5. Milk

Main food sources: batter, butter, cheese, cream, crème fraîche, ice cream, fromage frais, milk, yoghurt.

Main drink sources: beverages made with milk or milk powder.

Watch out for: bakery goods, breads, desserts, pancakes, puddings, sauces, sweets and many other processed and packaged foods.

Close relatives: other animal milks may cause reactions. A cross-reaction with beef is possible.

Label-reading tips: look for words containing 'casein', 'curd', 'lactose', 'lactalbumin', 'lactoglobulin', 'milk', 'Quark', 'whey'. The following do not contain milk and need not be avoided in a milk-free diet: 'lactate', 'lactic acid', 'lactitol', 'lactone', 'lactylate'. 'Dairy free' should really only refer to products free from cow's milk so 'dairy free' does not necessarily include other animal milks, but it may do. 'Suitable for vegans' is a term likely to be more reliable as it should mean completely free of all animal milks and products.

Related risks (non-food): some medicines and homeopathic remedies and 'tissue salts' contain lactose (milk sugar) as a filler. This should not cause a problem if the sensitivity is to milk protein (casein). (Ask your pharmacist or doctor about obtaining medication that is not blended with lactose.) Components of milk may be found in dishwasher powder and washing-up liquid (so rinse well), furniture polish and toothpaste.

Foods to have instead:

Milk: try other animal milks such as goat's, sheep or buffalo. There are several non-animal 'milk' alternatives including soya, rice, oat, almond (and other nut and seed milks) and pea-based milk. Fruit or vegetable juices may be suitable alternatives on occasions. As animal milks are a good source of calcium, choose a calcium-enriched alternative *(see 'Milks Alternative' table in Chapter 11),* make sure you eat plenty of foods containing calcium (and its partner-mineral magnesium) such as fish, leafy green vegetables, nuts and whole grains and/or take a nutritional supplement containing calcium. Not all milk alternatives are suitable for babies and young children so check with a health-care professional first.

Yoghurt: try yoghurt made from other animal milks such as goats and sheep. Soya-based yoghurts and desserts are also available. The rice dessert recipe in this handbook can provide a quick alternative dessert which can be enjoyed cold or hot.

Cheese: alternative 'cheeses' usually contain soya. Pâtés and dips (such as hummus) and tofu can be used in some meals to take the place of cheese.

Butter: milk-free margarines are available instead of butter, or use olive oil on bread and potatoes. Ghee or clarified butter may be tolerated by some milk-sensitive people.

Protein: other protein-containing foods such as meat, fish, beans and lentils can be used to substitute for the protein obtained from milk.

6. Oranges

Main food sources: orange fruit.

Main drink sources: orange juice, orange drinks.

Watch out for: orange lollies, sorbets, sweets, ice creams, some flavoured beers, some spirits and liqueurs.

Close relatives: lemon, grapefruit, lime.

Label-reading tips: usually listed as 'orange'; could be hidden as 'flavouring'.

Related risks (non-food): orange-coloured additives such as tartrazine (E102), the azo dye and yellow colouring, orange oil in environmentally-friendly paint thinners.

Foods to have instead: oranges are not the only fruit! Kiwi fruit are probably closest in texture and taste and are easily available.

7. Soya

Main food sources: miso, soya beans, soya cheese, soya flour, soya oil, soya meal, soya milk, soya noodles, soy sauce, soya yoghurt, TVP – 'textured vegetable protein', tamari, tempeh, tofu, 'vegetarian' products such as sausages, burgers and mince.

Main drink sources: some coffee substitutes, soups.

Watch out for: bakery products, meats, ice cream, desserts, sauces and many packaged and processed foods. Genetically-modified soya represents an unknown risk which is a concern for many people.

Close relatives: a sensitivity to other members of the legume (bean) family *(see 'Food Families' table in this chapter)* which includes peanuts, is possible.

Label-reading tips: look out for 'vegetable', 'TVP' – 'textured vegetable protein'. Lecithin (E322) is usually soya-derived. 'Contains genetically-modified ingredients' may refer to soya.

Related risks (non-food): breast implants made from soya instead of silicone may cause problems in some people. Some varnishes, paints, inks, papers, plastics.

Foods to have instead: packaged and processed foods that are free from soya. Toasted sesame or hemp oil can be used instead of soy sauce. Vegetarians or vegans relying on soya products as their main protein source will need to obtain protein from other legumes, nuts and seeds. Quorn (a mushroom-based meat substitute containing egg) may be acceptable.

8. Tomatoes

Main food sources: baked beans, casseroles, ketchup, tomato sauce, tomato soup, tomato salad.

Main drink sources: tomato juice and cocktails such as 'Bloody Mary' which contain tomato juice.

Watch out for: meat dishes, sauces, stews, soups and other packaged and processed foods.

Close relatives: other members of the nightshade family *(see 'Food Families' table in this chapter).*

Label-reading tips: usually listed as 'tomato'.

Related risks (non-food): medication that contains atropine, belladonna and scopolamine.

Foods to have instead: try pesto pasta sauce (made from basil and pinenuts) with lima (butter) beans instead of 'baked beans'. Use chicken, miso or vegetable stock instead of tinned tomatoes in soups, stews and casseroles.

9. Wheat

Main food sources: most batters, biscuits, breads, cakes, chapattis, naan bread, pasta, pastry, pitta bread, pizza base, some poppadoms.

Main drink sources: ale, beer, gin, lager, malt, malted milk drinks, spirits, whisky.

Watch out for: bakery products, baking powder, breadcrumbs, breakfast cereals, burgers, confectionery, crackers, croutons, dumplings, flour, gravy, noodles, pancakes, puddings, pretzels, rye bread (may contain wheatflour), sauces, sausages, stuffing mix, snackfoods, soups, spices (to prevent clumping), waffles and many packaged and processed foods.

Close relatives: bulgar wheat, couscous, durum wheat, kamut, semolina, spelt and triticale are all types of wheat that are likely to cause symptoms in a wheat-sensitive person. Despite its name, buckwheat is not related to wheat. It is a member of the same family as rhubarb and not a member of the grass family. If gluten in wheat is the problem, a cross-reaction with other gluten-containing grains is likely *(see 'Cross-reactions' section in this chapter)*.

Label-reading tips: apart from 'wheat', check for words including 'bran', 'cereal', 'farina', 'gluten', 'flour', 'malt', 'MSG', 'plant/vegetable protein/gum', 'rusk', 'starch' – these may all contain wheat.

Related risks (non-food): glue on labels, stamps, envelopes etc. (spit, don't lick!), communion wafers, some medications, playdough.

Foods to have instead: alternatives to wheat-based bread include breads made from rye including pumpernickel bread or corn (maize) bread. Non-wheat crackers can substitute for bread and include rice cakes, oat cakes, Ryvita and corn crackers. Other non-wheat flours suitable for making batters or baking include buckwheat, chestnut, chickpea (gram), lupin, millet, potato, rice, sago, soya, tapioca. Wheat-free baking powder is available. Oats can be used for crumbles, biscuits and flapjacks. Note that gluten-free products are not necessarily wheat-free.

10. Yeast

It is almost impossible to avoid yeast completely. It is more a question of reducing the main sources.

Main food sources: all leavened bread, most bakery products. Also cheese, dried fruits, fermented foods, malt (made by fermenting grains with yeast), meat extracts and meat products, nuts (unless freshly shelled), pâtés, stock cubes, vinegar, yeast extract and spread (e.g. Marmite, Vegemite). Any food that is not fresh or which may be mouldy.

Main drink sources: alcoholic drinks. Beer and wine contain high levels. Distilled spirits contain much less. Citrus fruit juices (unless freshly squeezed), ginger ale and beer, malted drinks. Black tea.

Watch out for: condiments such as dressings, pickles, sauces, spreads.

Close relatives: moulds and mushrooms, truffles and other members of the fungus family.

Label-reading tips: 'yeast' is the obvious clue but yeasts found on dried fruit or nuts won't be listed. Also look out for 'hydrolysed vegetable protein' or 'leavening'. Citric acid and MSG (monosodium glutamate) may be derived from yeast. Quorn (a mushroom-based meat substitute) may cause problems.

Related risks (non-food): nutritional supplements (especially B-vitamins) unless labelled as yeast-free. Some medications such as antibiotics and penicillin. Yeasts and moulds in the environment and particularly associated with damp environments.

Foods to have instead: unleavened bread such as pitta bread, chapatis, parathas. Also soda bread and sourdough breads which are leavened without adding yeast. Yeast is a good source of B-vitamins which can be obtained from other food sources such as avocados, bananas, whole grains, nuts, seeds, beans, meat and fish. Distilled vinegar may be tolerated.

Cross-reactions

Cross reactions can occur between members of the same food family or other foods which, because of other similarities, can be thought of as close relatives. However, unless you have a potentially life-threatening, 'classical' allergy to a food (where it is essential to avoid related foods), it is worth testing each individual food separately as you may not necessarily be sensitive to all – or indeed any – close relatives.

Cross-reactions between Foods

Animal Milks

If you react to cow's milk you may also have a sensitivity to other animal milks such as goat, sheep or buffalo milks. If your sensitivity to cow's milk is fairly minor it can be worth trying out these other animal milks.

Eggs

Cross-reactions may occur between eggs from different birds such as hen, goose, duck, quail.

Fish and Shellfish

Cross-reactions between different fish and also shellfish (crustaceans) and molluscs (such as mussels) are more likely in the case of classical allergic reactions but do not necessarily follow with other types of sensitivity.

Gluten-containing Grains

If gluten sensitivity is the reason behind a sensitivity to wheat (for example) then it is likely that rye, barley and oats, which also contain gluten, will provoke symptoms.

Nuts

Although peanuts are a legume (and not a nut) they are included in the nut group when investigating sensitivities. Note that arachis oil is from peanuts and it can be found in some skin products.

Reactions to foods can also be triggered through a cross-reaction with non-food substances in the environment, such as pollens or latex.

Rotation, Rotation, Rotation

A rotation way of eating can evolve naturally as you discover more alternative foods that you enjoy or, if you prefer, it can be planned from the start.

A rotation diet is a way of eating that can have several benefits.

- ♣ A rotation diet can improve how you feel. Just by spreading out the variety of foods that you eat over several days, this can be all you need to reduce the 'total load' of food stressors on your body and experience benefits to health.
- ♣ A rotation diet can be used to investigate the effects of a suspect food. The influence of a food on your emotional or mental health can become more obvious when you are not eating it every day.
- ♣ A rotation diet can be used to manage multiple food sensitivities. If you find that you are sensitive to a lot of foods, and don't want to restrict your diet by cutting out all the foods that cause you problems, then a rotation diet can provide a way forward.
- ♣ A rotation diet can reduce the risk of developing new food sensitivities in the future. This is because a rotation diet avoids overloading the body with any one particular food.

A rotation diet means you reduce the amount you eat of a food by eating it on some days and not others. The more days you can leave in between having the food and the next time you eat it, the better. Whilst it is easier to start with a two-day rotation (*see Chapter 5*), the best type of rotation diet to work towards is at least a four-day rotation of foods. This is where you leave three clear days before you eat the food again. If it is easier to plan, you could extend the four-day rotation diet to a 'once-a-week' rotation diet, where you eat a food just once every seven days, such as only at the weekend.

People living alone who may end up with 'left-over' food that could go to waste (and which can't be frozen) may choose to plan a slightly different type of rotation diet. To avoid having to throw away perfectly good food, each day of the rotation diet is immediately repeated. This means that the same food is eaten for two days in succession and then six days are left clear before eating it again.

Instead of trying to rotate everything you eat, you may find it easier to rotate some foods only. Even the most carefully planned rotation diet cannot take into account unexpected events, so be prepared to treat any hiccups in your special diet philosophically. The section on slip-ups provides some tips for how to deal with unexpected changes to your chosen diet.

A rotation way of eating can evolve naturally as you discover more alternative foods that you enjoy or, if you prefer, it can be planned from the start. Although some books do provide ready-made rotation diets, planning your own gives you the opportunity to tailor it to your particular preferences and needs. The following are the steps you need to follow to plan a four-day rotation diet to suit your tastes and lifestyle – the example provided will clarify the process.

Planning a Rotation Diet

1   Take a large sheet of paper and draw a grid as in the example below. The grid will need to include a single column to contain the different food groups (as described in Chapter 3) so that you can check you are planning a balanced diet. The food groups you need to include are starchy foods, fruit and vegetables, meat/fish (or vegetarian alternatives for these), milk and dairy foods (or non-milk/dairy substitutes) and foods containing fats, oils and sugar.

2   You will also need columns for each day of the rotation diet you are planning. The number of days you include may be determined by the number of alternatives you will be able to get hold of easily. Without giving consideration to the practicalities of sustaining a rotation diet, it will be much more difficult to make it work. Therefore it is important to be realistic about what you can manage.

3   Under each food group heading, list the foods you could eat in this category of food. This list will contain any suspect foods you want to investigate through a rotation diet. Include known culprit foods you are only mildly sensitive to, if that's what you have decided to do; otherwise leave them out of your list. Be honest about how easy it will be for you to sustain the changes that you are planning, and limit yourself to those foods that you know you can obtain and which you will want to eat.

4   Have an additional column as a 'spare' day. This allows you more choice and flexibility within the rotation of foods so that you can deal with unexpected events without necessarily having to 'slip up' on your diet. The foods allocated to the 'spare' day can be swapped with, or added to, the foods that have already been allocated to a particular day.

5   Allocate a different food from your list of alternatives to each day of your rotation plan.

6   Any foods listed in the first column that you haven't allocated to a particular day can be allocated to the 'spare' day.

7   The remainder of your diet can be made up from foods that you are not rotating and can be thought of as a 'free choice' category.

Evolving a Simple Rotation Diet

Let us consider the example of Sarah. Sarah wanted to avoid wheat and cow's milk completely for a while as she found that she felt much better when she eliminated these from her daily diet. To keep her diet nutritionally balanced and as varied and interesting as possible, she wished to include as many alternatives to wheat and cow's milk as she could. All other foods she thought of as a 'free choice' which she could eat freely. Sarah wanted to reduce the risk of developing any new sensitivities, so she also followed the general guideline of having a variety of foods spread across several days.

Following the steps given above, this is the meal plan that Sara came up with.

Food group	Day 1	Day 2	Day 3	Day 4	Spare foods
1. Starchy Foods					
Choose between:	rice	corn	buckwheat	oats	millet
buckwheat					sweet potato
corn					yam
millet					white potato
oats					
rice					
rye					
quinoa					
sweet potato					
white potato					
yam					

2. Fruit and Vegetables

Free choice

3. Meat, Fish and Vegetarian Substitutes

Free choice

continued...

4. Milk and Dairy Foods (or Non-milk and Dairy Substitutes)

Choose between:	rice	almond	soya	oat	goat's milk
almond milk					sheep milk
goat's milk					pea milk
oat milk					
rice milk					
sheep milk					
soya milk					
pea milk					

5. Foods Containing Fat, Oils and Sugar

Free choice

Because Sarah was rotating two sets of alternative foods, she had to make sure she allocated the same type of ingredient to the same day. In this example rice, as well as milk made from rice, were therefore allocated to the same day – a 'rice day'. Similarly, oats as well as milk made from oats were both allocated to another day – an 'oat day'.

Sarah then used the rotation diet she had drawn up to help her list meals she could have on each day.

Planning Meals from the Rotation Diet

When planning what to eat, Sarah found it helpful to think of each day according to the main food she was rotating. So one day was thought of as a 'rice-based day', for example, and another as a 'corn-based day'.

Meal	Day 1	Day 2	Day 3	Day 4
Breakfast	Rice porridge	Cornflakes	Pancakes made from soya/buckwheat/ chickpea/millet flour	Oat Porridge
	rice milk	almond milk	soya milk	oat milk
	+ free choice such as fresh fruit/dried fruit/nuts			
Lunch	rice noodles	corn crackers	buckwheat noodles	oat cakes
	+ free choice			
Dinner	rice	polenta (from corn)	buckwheat pasta	sweet potato
	+ free choice			
Snacks	rice cakes	corn crisps popcorn	Ryvita	oat cakes oat flapjack
	+ free choice			

Grilled Sardines on Corn/Maize Bread

Type:	Quick lunch or supper
Equipment:	Small bread tin, oven, grill/broiler, grinder for linseeds (optional)
Preparation time:	10 mins (bread), 1 min (grilled sardines)
Cooking time:	45 mins (bread), 5 mins (grilled sardines)

Corn/maize bread can make a good alternative for those sensitive to wheat and rye-based bread which both contain gluten. If you don't wish to make your own then corn/maize bread can be purchased from most health-food stores. This recipe is for sourdough bread which does not use yeast. It is therefore suitable for those avoiding yeast and its texture is closer to that of cake than traditional leavened breads. There is also the option to add linseeds which are the main vegetarian source of omega-3 oils and also provide useful fibre or 'roughage'. Tinned sardines, which are readily available and inexpensive to buy, can be used for this recipe. They are also an excellent source of omega-3 oils, the essential good mood nutrient.

Ingredients (per person)

For the grilled sardines:
1 small tin sardines in olive oil, spring water or brine

For the corn/maize bread (serves 4):
150g/6oz/1½ cups corn/maize meal or corn/maize flour
150g/6oz/1½ cups rice flour
50g/2oz/½ cup ground/whole linseeds (optional)
1 tbsp mixed dried herbs (optional)
pinch (sea) salt
1 tsp sodium or potassium bicarbonate
300ml/½ pint/1 cup rice milk

Method

To make the corn/maize bread:

1   Preheat the oven to 180°C/350°F/Gas Mark 4.
2   Mix together the dry ingredients.
3   Make a 'well' in the middle and pour in half the rice milk.
4   Stir together and keep adding the remainder of the milk until the ingredients stick together to form a single lump (you may want to use your hands for this). You may need slightly less or more milk than given in the ingredients list.
5   Bake for 45 mins approx.
6   When ready, remove from oven. If necessary, loosen edges with spatula or fish slice and tip out of tin to cool, preferably on a wire rack.

Ready?	Sticking a clean knife into the centre of the bread is a good way of testing whether or not the bread is ready.
Underdone	Knife comes out very sticky, bread still soft to touch and outside no darker in colour.
Just right	Knife comes out virtually clean, bread firm to touch and outside slightly brown.
Overdone	Knife comes out clean, bread feels hard and outside is beginning to burn.
Trouble-shooting tips	Bread mix too runny to form a ball of dough: try adding more corn/maize meal and rice flour in equal amounts. Even runny doughs usually work out alright in this recipe. Overdone bread: don't worry, it'll probably still make great toast.

Method

To make the grilled sardines on corn/maize bread:

1   Toast the corn/maize bread under the grill. (This is because it can be quite crumbly and is more likely to break up in a toaster.)
2   Open the tin of sardines and drain excess liquid.
3   Place in a bowl and mash with a fork. Any bones you find are usually soft enough to eat and make a good source of calcium, but can be lifted out if you prefer.
4   Pile mashed fish onto toast (no need for butter or margarine) and squash down with fork.
5   Place under grill for approx. 5 mins.

Ready?

Underdone	Fish is cool and looks no different to when you put it under the grill.
Just right	Fish beginning to 'sizzle' and look a darker colour.
Overdone	The fish and any exposed edges of the bread are burning.

Continuing Your Investigations

Women may find that their food sensitivities are increased during the latter part of their menstrual cycle.

Your sensitivity to any one food is likely to be influenced by the other stressors in your 'total load'. Your total load, which was described in Chapter 1, includes the idea of a threshold of tolerance which, if exceeded, leads to symptoms being produced. Anything you find overly stressful can contribute to your total load, and managing all the things that you know you find difficult can be quite an art. This idea of the total load can explain why sometimes you can 'get away with' eating a food that sometimes makes you feel bad and other times it proves to be the 'last straw'.

Physical symptoms of irritable bowel syndrome (IBS), for example, such as diarrhoea and constipation, often become worse during stressful times. In addition, many sufferers of this condition have found that certain foods are also associated with these symptoms. One way to manage IBS is to become aware of the situations *and* the foods that are sources of stress, and then to take steps to prevent them occurring together. This helps reduce the total load of stressors being experienced at any one time.

Women may find that their food sensitivities are increased during the latter part of their menstrual cycle. In the two weeks before their period, they may not be able to tolerate foods that, at other times of their cycle, they can eat without any problem. It is worth being aware of non-food-related events that can contribute to your sensitivity. This information will be extremely useful as you plan your investigations and manage your sensitivities.

Having investigated your list of suspect foods to reveal which were the culprits guilty of making you feel worse should you eat them, you may now be wondering if there are any other possible culprit foods lurking in your diet. If your health has improved sufficiently as a result of the changes you have already made then there is probably no need to take your investigations further. If, however, there are odd occasions when you feel worse for no apparent reason, you may like to consider something you ate as being a possible explanation.

If you are feeling worse after eating something you don't usually have then it is reasonable to suspect the novel food. Alternatively, it may be that a bit more detective work is needed to unravel the mystery of what is affecting you and why.

Natural Chemicals

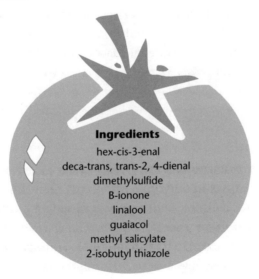

Ingredients
hex-cis-3-enal
deca-trans, trans-2, 4-dienal
dimethylsulfide
B-ionone
linalool
guaiacol
methyl salicylate
2-isobutyl thiazole

Fig 18 – Natural chemicals in a tomato

'Natural' doesn't mean 'chemical-free', for even completely unadulterated food contains chemicals. But the combination of chemicals found naturally in foods is generally less problematic than the individual artificial chemicals that can be added to food. Nevertheless, some food effects can be due to natural substances causing symptoms in sensitive people. Sometimes links emerge between a culprit food that you know upsets you and closely related suspect foods. The following food groupings may provide some interesting 'leads' to guide your inquiries. In the lists below a food may be found under more than one heading. Where there are possible links with artificial additives (such as synthetic versions of the naturally occurring substance), these are also given.

Food Detective Story

Whilst out walking one sunny Sunday afternoon, Paul and his girlfriend decided to visit a local pub for a refreshing drink. They weren't drinking alcohol that day so chose to have some ginger beer instead. Soon after drinking the ginger beer, Paul started to feel, as he described it, 'funny in the head'. The sensation, difficult to put into words, was as if his thinking processes had slowed down and his brain had become 'fuzzy' like 'cotton wool'. Aware of the risks of certain artificial additives in foods and drinks, he checked the label on the bottle. The only suspect was 'something called benzoic acid', which Paul hadn't noticed before as causing him a problem.

Later that weekend, Paul and his girlfriend were doing some baking. He opened a jar of cinnamon powder and smelt the aroma. He immediately had a 'brain numbing' sensation similar to the one he had experienced after drinking the ginger beer. Fortunately, this disappeared after about 30 minutes. Wondering if the cinnamon and ginger beer substances were somehow linked, Paul decided to do some detective work.

His inquiries uncovered an unexpected link between the cinnamon and the artificial additive benzoic acid (E210) that was in the ginger beer. Commonly used as a preservative, benzoic acid is a synthetic form of a naturally occurring group of chemicals called benzoates, found in cinnamon. Both artificial and natural forms of benzoate can cause reactions in some people.

Paul now chooses to avoid ginger beer that contains benzoic acid and also foods containing cinnamon. He is in the process of testing his reaction to other naturally high-benzoate-containing foods. 'It was very reassuring,' he said, 'to learn that there is a logical explanation for the two, apparently unrelated, food reactions.' (A list of naturally occurring benzoates can be found later in this chapter.)

Amines in Food

Amines can occur naturally in food as well as in the brain and body. Some naturally occurring amines that may provoke symptoms can be found in the foods listed below. The levels of amines found naturally in foods vary. These lists are intended as a guide only.

Histamine

Foods can contain naturally occurring histamine or may stimulate the release of histamine in the body. Histamine is also formed in food by the action of certain bacteria. These foods include:

aubergine (eggplant)

beer

cheese

chocolate

egg white (raw)

fermented foods (e.g. soya products,
    sauerkraut)

some fish

pumpkin

some sausages (e.g. pepperoni, salami,
    bologna)

shellfish

spinach

strawberries

tea

tomatoes

vinegar

wine

Related Risks: azo dyes (e.g. tartrazine), benzoates, BHA (butylated hydroxyanisole) and BHT (butylated hydoxytoluene), some cosmetics and toiletries and naturally occurring benzoates. **Histamine** is also an important brain chemical which is involved in the immune system and allergic reactions. Both too much and insufficient histamine have been associated with mental health problems (see Chapter 3).

Serotonin (5-hydroxytryptamine)

Serotonin can be found in:

avocados

bananas

pineapples

plantain

plums

tomatoes

molluscs (e.g. octopus, mussels)

Phenylethylamine

Phenylethylamine is found at high levels in the following foods:

several cheeses	red wine
chocolate	

Tyramine

Tyramine is present in a number of foods, particularly in:

aubergines (eggplants)	red plums
avocados	salted, smoked or pickled fish
bananas	(especially pickled herring)
broad (fava) beans	some sausages (such as bologna,
(most) cheeses	pepperoni and salami)
chicken liver	sour cream
fermented drinks	tomatoes
fermented soya bean extract	vinegar (and pickles)
meat extract (e.g. Bovril, Oxo)	wine (especially red)
peanuts	yeast extract (e.g. Marmite, Vegemite)
raspberries	

Related Risks: as the action of bacteria on protein produces tyramine, stale food or food which may be 'going off' and game meats will contain higher amounts of this substance.

Tyramine Sensitivity is caused by a fault in the monoamine oxidase enzyme system that normally breaks down tyramine. Symptoms include hot and itchy feelings, sweating and lightheadedness. Severe tyramine sensitivity can cause dangerous rises in blood pressure which may be signalled by a throbbing headache. The MAOI (monoamine oxidase inhibitor) type of antidepressant can interact with naturally occurring tyramine in food. Foods containing particularly high levels of tyramine must be avoided when on this type of medication.

Benzoates in Food

At very high concentrations, benzoates may have a narcotic affect (depressing brain function). Benzoic acid occurs naturally in foods at varying levels and is particularly high in the following:

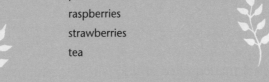

anise

cinnamon

cloves

cranberries

nutmeg

prunes

raspberries

strawberries

tea

Synthetic Benzoates: these are a common ingredient in many flavourings and can be used as a preservative in processed foods and also as a bleaching agent. Benzoates can also be found in non-food items such as the ice used for keeping fish cool at the fishmonger's, in toothpaste and toiletries. PABA (para-aminobenzoic acid), for example, is found in many sunscreen lotions.

Label Check: any words containing the following – benzoic acid, sodium benzoate, benzyl, benzoyl.

Related Risks: if you are sensitive to aspirin (acetylsalicylic acid), consider also the possibility of a sensitivity to benzoates.

Lectins in Food

Lectins are a naturally occurring toxin found in a lot of foods and are particularly high in legumes or pulses. Many lectins are inactivated by cooking but can still cause symptoms in some people. There is a special diet which associates certain blood types with different lectins in food. Apparently blood-group specific lectins can bind with blood and tissue cells and cause damage within the body.

Phenols in Food

Phenols in food are impossible to avoid entirely. They are found in both natural and synthetic food colourings and have been associated with migraine and autism. Foods higher in phenols include:

apple juice   cranberries
bananas   herbs
buckwheat   mango
cherries   peas
chocolate   rhubarb
citrus fruit

Related Risks: paracetamol

Salicylates in Food

Salicylates are naturally occurring, aspirin-like chemicals that have been associated with hyperactivity. Salicylates are found in many foods in varying amounts. They are likely to be at higher levels in the following:

almonds

apples (sharp tasting such as Granny Smith's)

Benedictine liqueur

berries

broccoli

cherries

chicory

citrus fruit (oranges etc.)

Drambuie liqueur

dried fruit

endive

gherkins

grapes

guavas

herbs

kiwi fruit

liquorice

macadamia nuts

mint, peppermint

mushrooms

peppers

pineapples

pinenuts

pistachio nuts

port

radishes

raspberries

rum

spices

tea

Tia Maria liqueur

tomatoes

watercress

Worcestershire sauce

Wintergreen oil

Related Risks: a sensitivity to aspirin (acetylsalicylic acid) is likely if you are sensitive to naturally occurring salicylates. Also, cigarettes and toiletries flavoured with mint, menthol and wintergreen. If you are sensitive to salicylates it is worth also checking for reactions to artificial additives including the azo dye tartrazine (E102), sulphites and also synthetic and naturally occurring benzoates.

Label Check: look for words containing 'salicylic acid' or 'salicylate' and 'menthol'.

Foods in Alcoholic Drinks

♣ This table gives a general guide to the common culprit foods found in alcoholic drinks but ingredients do vary between different brands and types within any category.

♣ All alcoholic drinks contain yeast, but the distilled spirits will contain considerably less than wines and beers.

♣ Rum and tequila make the best choice for an alcoholic drink in terms of the low risk from common culprit foods.

	barley	citrus	corn	oats	rye	wheat	yeast
ale/beer	✓		✓				✓
brandy							✓
gin	✓	✓	✓	✓	✓		✓
rum							✓
tequila							✓
liqueurs	✓	✓	✓				✓
whisky	✓		✓	✓	✓	✓	✓
vodka	✓		✓		✓	✓	✓
wine			✓				✓

✓ = usually found

Food Families

The members of a food family can be sufficiently alike so that if you are sensitive to one member of the family you may 'cross-react' and have a sensitivity to some of its close relatives.

Food can be grouped into families. The members of a food family can be sufficiently alike so that if you are sensitive to one member of the family you may 'cross-react' and have a sensitivity to some of its close relatives. Although food families can provide a fruitful line of inquiry, be aware of the power of expectation (*see Chapter 9*), keep an open mind and test each food individually.

Fruit and Vegetables

AMARANTH
Amaranth

APPLE
Apple
Crab-apple
Pear
Pectin
Quince
Rosehip

ARROWROOT
Arrowroot

ASTER
Artichoke (globe &
    Jerusalem)
Burdock
Chamomile
Chicory
Dandelion
Endive
Escarole
Lettuce
Romaine
Safflower
Salsify
Sunflower (seeds/oil)
Tarragon
Yarrow

BANANA
Banana
Cardamom

Ginger
Plantain
Turmeric

BEECH
Beechnut
Chestnut

BEET
Beetroot
Chard
Spinach
Sugar beet

BIRCH
Hazelnuts/Filberts

BRAZIL
Brazilnut

BUCKWHEAT
Buckwheat
Rhubarb
Sorrel

CAPER
Caper

CARROT
Angelica
Aniseed
Caraway
Carrots
Celeriac

Celery
Chervil
Coriander
Comfrey
Cumin
Dill
Fennel
Parsley
Parsnips
Samphire

CASAVA
Casava/Tapioca

CASHEW
Cashew
Mango
Pistachio

CITRUS
Citron
Clementine
Grapefruit
Kumquat
Lemon
Lime
Mandarin
Orange
Satsuma
Tangerine
Ugly

CONIFER
Pine nut

ELDERBERRY
Elderberry

FLAXSEED
Flaxseed/Linseed

FUNGI
Mushroom
Truffle
Yeast (baker's/brewer's)

GOOSEBERRY
Blackcurrant
Gooseberry
Redcurrant

GRAPE
Grape/Currant/Sultana/Raisin
Tartar (cream of)

GRASS
Bamboo shoots
Barley
Corn (maize)
Malt
Millet
Oats
Rice
Rye
Sugar cane/Molasses
Sorghum
Wheat

HEATHER
Bilberry
Blueberry

Cranberry
Huckleberry
Sloe
Wintergreen

HEMP
Hemp seeds/oil

KIWI
Kiwi

LAUREL
Avocado
Bayleaf
Cassia buds/bark
Cinnamon
Sassafras

LEGUME
Alfalfa
Black-eyed pea
Butterbean
Beansprouts
Carob
Chickpea/Garbanzo
Fenugreek
French bean/Green bean
Haricot beans
Kidney bean
Lentil
Lima bean
Liquorice
Mung bean
Navy bean
Pinto bean
Peas

Peanuts
Senna
Soya bean
Wax bean

LILY
Asparagus
Chives
Garlic
Leek
Onion
Shallot

LYCHEE
Lychee

MACADAMIA
Macadamia nut

MADDER
Coffee

MALLOW
Cottonseed
Hibiscus
Okra

MAPLE
Maple syrup

MELON
Cantaloupe
Cucumber
Courgette/Zucchini
Gherkin
Marrow

Melon (honeydew)
Pumpkin
Squash
Watermelon

MINT
Balm
Basil
Bergamot
Catnip
Horehound
Lavender
Lemonbalm
Marjoram
Mint
Oregano
Peppermint
Rosemary
Sage
Savory
Spearmint
Thyme

MORNING GLORY
Sweet potato

MULBERRY
Breadfruit
Fig
Hop
Mulberry

MUSTARD
Broccoli
Brussels sprout
Cabbage

Cauliflower
Chinese cabbage/leaves
Collards
Cress
Horseradish
Kale
Kohlrabi
Mustard
Radish
Rape (seed)
Swede/ Rutabaga
Turnip
Watercress

MYRTLE
Allspice
Clove
Guava

NUTMEG
Mace
Nutmeg

OLIVE
Olive

ORCHID
Vanilla

PALM
Coconut
Date
Palm
Sago

PAPAYA
Papain/Papaya/Pawpaw

PASSION FRUIT
Passion fruit

PEPPER
Pepper (black/white)
Peppercorns

PERSIMMON
Persimmon/Kaki

PINEAPPLE
Pineapple

POMEGRANATE
Pomegranate
Grenadine

POTATO (NIGHTSHADE)
Aubergine/Eggplant
Cayenne
Chilli
Paprika
Peppers/Capsicums
  (red & green)
Pimento
Potato
Sesame/Tahini
Tobacco
Tomato

PLUM
Almond
Apricot

Cherry
Damson
Nectarine
Peach
Plum
Prune

POPPY
Poppy seeds

ROSE
Blackberry
Boysenberry
Dewberry
Loganberry
Raspberry
Strawberry

Youngberry

SESAME
Sesame/tahini

STAR FRUIT
Star fruit

STERICULA
Chocolate
Cocoa
Cola

TEA
Tea

TIGER NUT
Tiger nut

VERBENA
Lemon verbena

WALNUT
Butternut
Hickory nut
Pecan nut
Walnut

WATER CHESTNUT
Waterchestnut

YAM
Yam

Meat

BOVID
Beef
Buffalo
Cow
Cow's milk & products
Goat
Goat's milk & products
Lamb
Sheep's milk & products
Veal

DEER
Caribou
Elk
Moose

Reindeer
Venison

DOVE
Pigeon

DUCK
Duck
Goose

GROUSE
Grouse
Partridge

GUINEA FOWL
Guinea fowl

HARE
Hare
Rabbit

PHEASANT
Chicken
Chicken egg
Peafowl
Pheasant
Quail

SWINE
Pork

TURKEY
Turkey

Seafood

CRUSTACEAN
Crab
Crayfish
Lobster
Prawn
Shrimp

MOLLUSC
Abalone
Clam
Cockle
Mussel
Oyster

Scallop
Snail
Squid

OCTOPUS
Octopus

Fish

ANCHOVY
Anchovy

BASS
Bass
Perch (White)
Yellow bass

CODFISH
Cod/Cod liver oil
Coley
Haddock
Hake
Ling/Saith
Pollock

EEL
Eel

FLOUNDER
Dab
Flounder
Halibut
Plaice
Sole
Turbot

HERRING
Herring
Sardine
Pilchard
Rollmop
Shad

MACKEREL
Bonito
Mackerel
Skipjack
Tuna

Tunny

MULLET
Mullet

PORGY
Bream
Porgy

SCORPION FISH
Ocean perch
Rockfish

SEA BASS
Grouper
Sea bass

SEA CATFISH
Catfish

SKATE	PIKE	STURGEON
Skate (Ray)	Pickerel	Caviar
	Pike	Sturgeon
MINNOW		
Carp	**SALMON**	**SUNFISH**
Chub	Salmon	Black bass
	Trout	
PERCH		**WHITEFISH**
Perch (Yellow)	**SMELT**	Whitefish
Red snapper	Smelt	

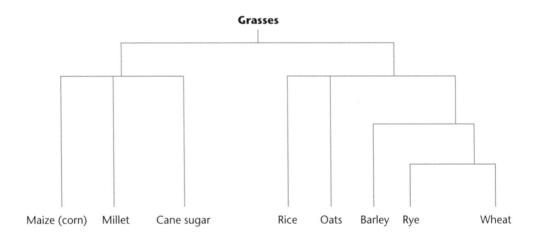

Fig 19 – The Grass Family Tree

Rye and wheat are closely-related members of the grass family and they contain the highest amounts of gluten.

Managing 'Slip-ups' and the Importance of Sustainability

Accept that until your new diet becomes fully integrated into your lifestyle, 'slip-ups' are inevitable.

Whatever the reasons behind the alterations you make to your diet, it is important that you are able to sustain the changes you make for as long as you want to. To do this you need to be realistic about your goals and appreciate the practical implications of a change in diet. Whilst short-term changes are easier to keep going, a permanent alteration to your diet can be difficult to sustain without considerable effort and commitment. To avoid disappointment it can be helpful to view bigger changes simply as goals you are working towards. Accept that until your new diet becomes fully integrated into your lifestyle, 'slip-ups' are inevitable.

Tricky times tend to include eating out where the availability of the alternatives you have come to rely on cannot be guaranteed. This is also when you can come up against considerable social pressures to eat foods that you have been carefully avoiding. It is worth considering how you might approach any slip-ups that do occur.

If you have been avoiding a food completely (or as part of a rotation diet) there will be occasions when, despite your best intentions, you will still manage to eat it. Perhaps you are out and about and there is simply no alternative, other than to go hungry. As this would risk a debilitating drop in blood-sugar levels, you may, reluctantly, decide that avoiding the food is no longer an option.

Another time it could be a special celebration that you want to enjoy but which, unfortunately, doesn't cater for your special dietary needs. Yet another possibility is that you eat something fully believing it to be free of whatever-it-is-you-are-avoiding. You then find out (perhaps by re-reading a food label or, prompted by your symptoms, you decide to ask someone) that a culprit food has in fact 'slipped through the net' and into your stomach. Of course, a 'slip-up' could be due to willpower which, at a time when you needed it most, decided to disappear altogether.

Whatever the reason behind a 'slip-up', it can be a particularly frustrating experience, especially if you know you are going to feel worse because of it. One way to deal with unplanned changes to your diet is to view them as an unexpected opportunity for you to gain some useful information.

From your 'slip up' you could learn, for example, how your body is getting on with improving its tolerance to the culprit food you have been avoiding. By adopting such an attitude, any occasion on which you inadvertently eat something you have been avoiding can be turned into the food 'challenge' that was explained in Chapter 5. When a 'slip-up' happens it is worth keeping an open mind as to the consequences, for you could be pleasantly surprised. You may find that your tolerance has improved and you now no longer need to be so careful to avoid the food completely.

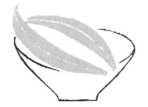

7

Caffeine and Chocolate

Occasionally the effect of a food means that it's easy to become involved in an addictive-type relationship with it.

Not all mind-altering drugs are illegal. A white crystalline powder in its purest form, this is probably the most widely used behaviour-modifying drug in the world. Openly consumed by adults for its ability to improve performance, mental ability and mood, children also enjoy it daily for the 'buzz' it provides. Addiction to this drug is common, with users needing frequent and regular 'top-ups' if they are to avoid unpleasant withdrawal symptoms. Should supplies of this substance be interrupted, addicts may suffer painful headaches that can last for days. But this is unlikely, for worldwide availability is firmly established with outlets that range from food store to drug store. The global industry which profits from its sale is worth millions, sources of the drug are widely publicized and it is government approved. The drug in question? It is caffeine.

This deliberately sensational description has been used to illustrate how many people use a familiar beverage and food to affect their mood. Whilst many food effects can be both beneficial and enjoyable, some food and drinks – rather like prescription drugs – can also produce some not-so-pleasant side-effects. Occasionally the effect of a food means that it's easy to become involved in an addictive-type relationship with it. Addictive substances are usually considered to be those that you need to take gradually more of in order to get the same effect, or those which cause withdrawal symptoms if you cut down on the amount you regularly consume.

Caffeine Chemistry

Caffeine is one of a group of chemicals called methylxanthines (two others are theophylline and theobromine) which are found naturally in tea leaves, coffee beans, cola nuts and cocoa beans. Caffeine is also found in over-the-counter medicines sold as painkillers and cold and flu remedies. Caffeine (and theobromine) stimulate the central nervous system, which is the brain and spinal cord, causing the heart to beat faster. The stimulatory effect of caffeine is likely due to its ability to block the absorption of a natural sedative in the brain called adenosine. By over-riding this natural sedative, caffeine fools the body to stay alert for longer.

The effects of caffeine are one example of the apparently addictive nature of some foods. Every time you have a cup of coffee or tea, a can of cola or chocolate drink or bar you will almost certainly be having some caffeine. Even so-called 'decaff' can, quite legitimately, contain small quantities of caffeine. An addictive-type relationship with a substance is not necessarily always unpleasant. As is the case with caffeine, the increased mental alertness and stimulation it appears to provide can be just what's needed. But the positive effects of consuming caffeine can be confused with the avoidance of caffeine-withdrawal symptoms. When this happens, an apparent benefit is merely the result of an 'addictive' need being satisfied. All that has been achieved is that the body has been prevented from entering an unpleasant caffeine withdrawal.

If you are a regular coffee drinker, the feelings of mental dullness and fatigue that caffeine appears to be so good at overcoming may be due to your body crying out for 'another hit'.

If, for example, you are a regular tea, coffee, cola or chocolate drinker (or eater), the feelings of mental dullness and fatigue (for example) that caffeine appears to be so good at overcoming may be due to your body crying out for 'another hit' of the caffeine it has become used to having so regularly. These symptoms can be signalling the start of a caffeine 'withdrawal' which, by having another intake of caffeine, you are managing to avoid. If you were to stick with your reduced caffeine consumption, you would find that after no more than a few days of 'clearing out your system' these unpleasant withdrawal symptoms would have disappeared (*see 'Coming off Caffeine' later in this chapter*).

Too much caffeine can cause anxiety, cravings, nervousness and depression.

Yet having a cup of coffee or tea also has a lot of positive psychological associations. We meet a friend for 'a coffee and a chat' or give ourselves a break by sitting down with a cup of tea. These things are very important but needn't be associated only with drinking coffee or tea. Unfortunately, the consumption of caffeine has its downside and too much of it (which is a different amount for each of us) can cause symptoms such as anxiety, cravings, nervousness and depression. The main concern with apparently addictive foods and drinks such as caffeine is that eating or drinking them every day puts the body under stress that, in the long term, can be damaging to mental and physical health (*see the explanation of the General Adaptation Syndrome in Chapter 1*).

When exploring the link between food and mood, caffeine consumption can be a good place to begin as it is a food that is relatively easy to spot in your diet. If you would like to look into your relationship with caffeine, you could start by seeing how much caffeine you are consuming on a regular basis. To do this you will need to know which are the foods and drinks that contain caffeine. So try this simple exercise that tests your existing knowledge and assumptions about the caffeine you consume.

Which Has Most?

Rank these in descending order of caffeine content, starting with the food or drink that contains the most caffeine:

- a cup of instant coffee
- a fizzy drink containing the herb guarana
- a cup of tea made with a tea bag
- a can of cola
- a cup of filter coffee
- a bar of plain chocolate
- a cup of 'hot chocolate'
- a bar of milk chocolate
- a cup of maté tea
- a cup of tea made with loose-leaf tea
- a cup of 'green' tea
- a cup of 'decaff'
- a cup of rooibos herbal tea
- a can of energy drink

Answer

As you might expect, **a cup of filter coffee** contains the most caffeine (the average mug contains around 100mg) then, in descending order:

- a can of energy drink
- instant coffee
- loose-leaf tea
- tea made with a bag (tea averages around 40mg caffeine per cup)
- green tea (a beneficial antioxidant, containing polyphenols – potent free-radical scavengers with some anti-carcinogenic action)
- cola (the average can contains around 23mg caffeine while some energy drinks have up to four times that amount)
- plain chocolate
- milk chocolate (plain chocolate has 40mg caffeine per 100g – nearly three times as much as milk chocolate)
- a cup of 'hot chocolate'
- a cup of 'decaff'
- a fizzy drink containing the herb guarana (a South American herb closely related to caffeine but possibly not as toxic)
- a cup of rooibos herbal tea (this is naturally caffeine-free although it does contain tannin, an 'antinutrient' which binds to minerals, such as iron and zinc, in the gut thus preventing their absorption)
- a cup of maté tea (a South American herbal drink containing matine, a central nervous system stimulant similar to caffeine but, it is claimed, without some of caffeine's negative effects. Maté is high in tannins)

Approximate Levels of Caffeine

♣ a cup of filter coffee	100mg
♣ a can of energy drink	80mg
♣ a cup of instant coffee	66mg
♣ a cup of tea made with loose-leaf tea	41mg
♣ a cup of tea made with a tea bag	40mg
♣ a can of cola	23mg
♣ a 50g bar of plain chocolate	20mg
♣ a 50g bar of milk chocolate	7mg
♣ a cup of 'hot chocolate'	5mg
♣ a cup of 'green' tea	4mg
♣ a cup of 'decaff'	3mg

Caffeine is also found in some painkillers, cold and flu remedies, diuretics, 'alertness' supplements, tonics and appetite suppressants.

Caffeine is also present in some over-the-counter medication such as painkillers (analgesics), cold and flu remedies, diuretics (to increase urine production), 'alertness' supplements, tonics and appetite suppressants. It can also be hidden in cola drinks and other food products listed as 'flavourings'.

The next step is for you to assess how much caffeine you are consuming on a regular basis. This is where your Food and Drink Diary will be very useful (*see Chapter 4*). In the next exercise, complete the table which lists the main sources of caffeine.

How Much Caffeine Do You Have?

Number of portions (i.e. cup/can/glass or small bar of chocolate) per day

Tea (including decaff)	_____	cups
Coffee (including decaff)	_____	cups
Chocolate (bars and other foods that contain chocolate and chocolate drinks)	_____	portions/cups
Cola (plus similar drinks)	_____	glasses/cans

Experiment by making changes and observing the effects of this change.

Your need for, and sensitivity to, caffeine will be different to the next person's, and ultimately only you can decide whether your intake is right for you. As a rough guide, having more than six cups of instant coffee a day is suggested as a comparatively 'high' level of consumption. But some people find that any amount of caffeine is too much for them to remain in good health. Your judgement will become more accurate once you have experimented by making changes to the amount you have and by observing the effects of this change. Guidance on the best way to do this is given later in this chapter. First, though, you may like to compare your level of caffeine consumption with a survey of 50 participants from the Food and Mood Project.

This table shows what percentage of Food and Mood Project participants drank cups of tea, coffee, cola (or other caffeine-containing fizzy drinks) or ate chocolate, together with the amount they consumed, measured as the number of portions per day. The survey was taken before the participants made any changes to their diet.

Caffeine Consumption Survey

Number of portions consumed per day

	0 zero	1–3 low	3–6 medium	6+ high
Tea (including decaff)	34%	47%	11%	8%
Coffee (including decaff)	29%	55%	10%	6%
Chocolate (bars and drink)	45%	50%	5%	0%
Cola (plus similar drinks)	55%	40%	5%	0%

- ♣ Taken as a group, most said they drank 1–3 cups of tea and between 1 and 3 cups of coffee per day (individuals may have drunk either tea or coffee and not both).
- ♣ Half of the participants surveyed said they ate at least one bar of chocolate or drank one cup of hot chocolate every day.
- ♣ Most said that they did not drink, on a regular basis, any cola or fizzy drinks containing caffeine.

Before you become too complacent (or overly concerned) about your level of caffeine consumption as compared to this survey, it is worth noting some facts about surveys. Many surveys – and this one is no exception – are not representative of the population as a whole. The people who took part in this survey were on Food and Mood Project courses they had chosen to attend. So we could assume that they were people who were already interested, and fairly motivated, in eating more healthily, compared with a genuine cross-section of the public. Also, what people say (when asked by a researcher for example) and what they actually do in private may be slightly (or even greatly) different. So, this type of information is best taken only as an indication of what other people are actually doing and used as a rough guide for comparison with our own patterns of behaviour.

Caffeine and Mood

Caffeine increases mental alertness and concentration and can improve performance. It can be useful and pleasurable to take. However, too much caffeine (and remember this will be a different amount for each person) has been found associated with:

- anxiety
- cravings
- depression
- emotional instability
- insomnia
- mood swings
- nervousness and 'jittery' feelings
- premenstrual syndrome (PMS)
- restlessness
- stress, including physical symptoms such as palpitations (rapid heart beat) and temporarily raised blood pressure.

A typical caffeine withdrawal picture is to have headaches first thing in the morning, fuzzy headedness or fatigue that is soon relieved by a morning cup of tea or coffee.

You can appear to be suffering from not having enough caffeine when symptoms such as irritability and poor concentration improve after you have had a caffeine-containing drink or snack. But if you are a regular caffeine user (irrespective of the quantity you have), these symptoms can also be caused by the start of a caffeine withdrawal (*see below*). The clue to look out for here are symptoms that disappear when you have caffeine. A typical caffeine withdrawal picture is to have headaches first thing in the morning, fuzzy headedness or fatigue that is soon relieved by a morning cup of tea or coffee. As we sleep our bodies begin to detoxify from the caffeine we have consumed the previous day so we may awake suffering withdrawal symptoms. These are quickly improved if we have some caffeine.

Case Study: Anxiety

Picture the scene: I'm on a busy tube train; I have a lot more stations to go before I reach my destination but I have to get off the train and I have to get off NOW. I can hardly breathe and I'm not sure where I am; I just know I need to get away from all the people around me.

Panic attacks were part of my day; they happened frequently and without warning and I couldn't seem to find a cure. I often had to desert my friends in a pub or club. I would leave restaurants before the main course had been served. As you can imagine, all this and sleepless nights as well led me to feel very anxious. At this time I rated my anxiety levels at 8 on a scale of 0–10. But all of that is now behind me.

I thought my problems were psychological but then I learned that most of my symptoms could be alleviated by cutting down on caffeine. I cut out coffee and reduced my intake of tea, replacing these with herbal teas and water. I could now give my anxiety levels a score of only 2 out of a possible 10.

Some months later I have now changed some of the foods that I eat, and instead of dairy foods I now have more soya products. I have also introduced more organic fruit and vegetables into my diet. Recently I have changed to eating foods that are wheat- and gluten-free and I find that I now sleep well and have lots more energy. And the panic attacks? They are a thing of the past.

Caffeine Quiz

Decide whether the following are true or false:

1   Caffeine is found in chocolate, tea, coffee and cola.

2   Caffeine is the most widely consumed stimulant drug in the world.

3   Caffeine can be bought in pills from the chemists.

4   Caffeine consumption is followed by an increase in blood pressure and adrenalin-production and can encourage glucose intolerance through its stimulatory effect on the adrenal glands.

5   Caffeine is absorbed quickly and stays in your body for about one hour.

6   If you're on the Pill, caffeine lasts longer in your body.

7   Drinking coffee could contribute to osteoporosis.

8   Caffeine is a diuretic (urine-producing) so if you drink too much you can become dehydrated.

9   Caffeine can make you constipated.

10   Caffeine can help with a hangover.

11   Drinking tea may contribute to becoming anaemic.

12   Caffeine taken on a regular basis can lead to addiction. This means you need to take more to get the same effect and suffer withdrawal symptoms if you stop taking it.

13   'Decaff' drinks mean all the caffeine has been taken out.

14   'Decaff' coffee can be made using dry-cleaning chemicals.

15   Too much caffeine can cause anxiety, nervousness and depression.

16   Not enough caffeine can make you irritable and have difficulty concentrating.

17   PMS can be helped by a caffeine-free diet.

18   Coming off caffeine 'cold turkey' takes three weeks.

19   You can treat caffeine withdrawal symptoms such as a headache by using the 'hair of the dog' approach, taking sips of coffee or tea.

20   Coffee enemas are sometimes used for treating cancer.

Answers

1   True.

2   True.

3   True: caffeine is found in painkillers and flu remedies.

4   True.

5   False: although caffeine is absorbed quickly and reaches peak levels in about an hour, it can remain the body for 2–12 hours.

6   True.

7   True: excessive caffeine consumption depletes the body's stores of calcium.

8   True.

9   True and False: coffee has a mild laxative effect but because of caffeine's diuretic effect it can contribute to constipation.

10   False: coffee may in fact aggravate a hangover by increasing dehydration due to its diuretic effect.

11   True: the consumption of tea or coffee within one hour of a meal has been shown to reduce iron absorption by up to 80 per cent.

12   True.

13   False: instant 'decaff' coffee must have no more than 0.3 per cent caffeine which means there can still be some caffeine in 'decaff'.

14   True: decaffeination can use an organic solvent such as methylene chloride or ethyl acetate which are also used in paint strippers, aerosols and dry-cleaning solutions. There is concern about the possibility of these solvent residues remaining in the decaffeinated product. Alternative methods use carbon dioxide or water.

15   True: these are symptoms of 'caffeinism'.

16   True: these are some symptoms of withdrawal from caffeine.

17   True: also, low fertility – a consumption of five mugs of coffee per day has been shown to produce a 60 per cent reduction in fertility.

18   False: the worst of the withdrawal symptoms are usually over after three to five days.

19   True: better still, drink plenty of water to help the detoxification process.

20   True: pioneered by the late Dr Gerson in the 1950s.

Fruity Flapjack

Type:	Snack
Equipment:	medium pan, hob, oven-proof dish/foil tray, oven
Preparation time:	5 mins
Cooking time:	40 mins

Flapjacks are a delicious and filling snack that can be carried easily when out and about to bridge the gap between meals. The oats that form the basis of this recipe are an excellent mood food for they are rich in B-vitamins and a good source of magnesium. They contain soluble fibre which is good for bowel-brain health. The honey or molasses (which also contain valuable nutrients) tend to have a lower GI than sugar and, when combined with the oats, will not raise blood sugar levels too high. Oats have a particularly low GI so these flapjacks won't start you off on a roller-coaster blood-sugar ride but will satisfy and keep you feeling good for longer.

Ingredients (serves 4)

100g/40oz/1 cup margarine (milk/dairy-free)

1 tbsp honey or black strap molasses

200g/8oz/2 cups oatflakes/rolled oats

25g/1oz/¼ cup walnut pieces

25g/1oz/¼ cup dried apricots (cut into small pieces)

Method

1   Preheat the oven to 180°C/350°F/Gas Mark 4.
2   Melt margarine in the pan over a low heat, add the honey and mix.
3   Add dry ingredients to pan and mix together well.
4   Put mixture into oven-proof dish so that it forms a layer about 2.5cm/1 inch thick. (Don't worry about any unused space – the mixture should be firm enough to stay at one end of a large dish.)
5   Press down firmly with the back of a large spoon.
6   Bake for approx. 30 mins.
7   Remove from oven and cut into pieces without removing from dish and then allow to cool.

Ready?

Underdone	Appears to be the same colour as uncooked mixture.
Just right	Slightly browner in colour.
Overdone	Starting to burn.

Trouble-shooting tip	Flapjacks too crumbly: use as a crunchy oat breakfast cereal or topping for fruit such as stewed apples. Next time you could try the following alterations: add slightly more margarine and/or honey/molasses; press the mixture down harder into the dish; powder half of the oatflakes in a liquidizer.

Chocolate and the Feel-good Factor

The pleasurable – and sometimes apparently addictive – effects of chocolate may be explained by its ability to affect brain chemicals or neurotransmitters that control mood, behaviour and mental functioning. As well as containing stimulatory methylxanthines described earlier, chocolate also contains phenylethylamine, or PEA. PEA (also found in red wine and some cheeses) can be produced in the body from phenylalanine, an amino acid found in protein foods.

The romantic associations we have with chocolate may be due to the effects on the brain of PEA which is understood to enhance endorphin levels, increase libido and act as a natural antidepressant. Sugar can also increase levels of the body's natural endorphins and chocolate bars often contain appreciable amounts of sugar. These mood-altering effects of chocolate may be why it is easy to become 'hooked on' it.

Caffeine Associations

The morning coffee with a friend, putting your feet up with a nice cup of tea, grabbing a cool refreshing can of cola, snuggling up to watch a film with a mug of cocoa and a packet of chocolate biscuits, or receiving a romantic box of chocolates are some of life's caffeine-associated pleasures. We have seen that the ingredients in these foods and drinks can have powerful effects on how we feel – which (of course) is often why we choose to have them! But what, do you feel, is in control – caffeine or you? Addictions to food are often not considered to be 'real addictions' or taken as seriously as addictive relationships with other substances such as alcohol or nicotine. But to the individuals concerned, a caffeine addiction can still be a disabling and distressing relationship with a substance that seems to have 'the upper hand'.

A caffeine addiction can be a disabling and distressing relationship with a substance that seems to have 'the upper hand'.

Quite apart from the real physiological effects of such foods, there are important psychological and social factors that come into play when we are deciding what to eat and drink. The diagram below gives some associations people make with coffee, tea or chocolate, based on work done by Food and Mood Project participants. Which of these do you relate to, and can you think of any others?

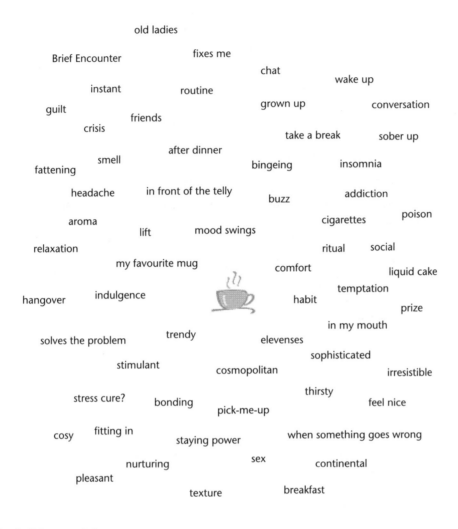

Fig 20 – Caffeine associations

Is Caffeine a Problem?

It is possible that some aspects of your health which you'd like to be different – perhaps anxiety, depression, mood swings, cravings, PMS – could be helped by cutting down on or coming off caffeine. Finding out for yourself by making changes and observing the effect of those changes is a way to take control and get valuable information that can't be obtained in any other way. Yet there are many reasons why we like to have coffee, tea, chocolate and cola drinks. Some of these are positive and some negative.

Being aware of reasons behind your food and drink choices creates a firm foundation for then changing what you do. If you are clearer about why you choose something you may be able to think of another way to gain the positive effects you need. You may have identified with some of the ideas in the diagram above or thought of some others that are special to you.

Consuming Caffeine

The next exercise asks you to try listing your reasons for drinking caffeine in two columns, one for 'positive' and the other for 'negative' reasons. It could look something like the example below:

+VE REASONS   -VE REASONS
e.g.   e.g.
it wakes me up in the morning   it keeps me awake at night
it keeps me going   it makes me irritable

Having listed the positive and negative reasons for doing something, you may find that you need more information before you know if you need to do anything about the caffeine in your diet. The only way to be certain of the effect that caffeine is having on *your* emotional and mental health is to cut down the amount you have (or even cut it out completely) and find out for yourself. You will then be in a better position to decide if, when and how you want to use this potent drug, based on your own experience.

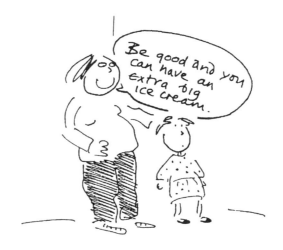

Coming off Caffeine

If you do decide to cut down or cut out caffeine, here are some hints to help you:

- Start by listing the sources of caffeine in your diet *(see previous pages)*.
- Work out how much you are consuming *(see previous pages)* and when.
- Think about the emotional and social reason why you might be consuming caffeine *(see above)* and how you could cater for these needs in other ways.
- Decide if you want to stop suddenly or wean yourself off gradually (if you stop suddenly you are likely to experience withdrawal symptoms for three to five days; if you wean yourself off gradually any withdrawal symptoms will be lessened).
- Stock up on alternative drinks *(see 'Caffeine Alternatives and Substitutes Survey' below)* and have a go!

Caffeine-withdrawal Symptoms

These are caused by the body detoxifying or 'getting rid' of the traces of caffeine in your body. Your brain also needs time to readjust to functioning without a regular dose of caffeine. For example, as you reduce the amount of caffeine you take, the 'receptor sites' in your brain which were previously taken up with caffeine become available to receive adenosine instead, the natural sedative whose absorption was previously being 'blocked' by the caffeine. As a result you may feel more sleepy and lethargic for the first few days as more of the natural sedative is being absorbed by your brain. This feeling may continue for a few days until your brain rebalances itself by closing down (or 'down-regulating') some of the receptor sites, so that you don't absorb as much adenosine and then don't feel as tired.

Withdrawal symptoms can be difficult to deal with so, if you are choosing to go 'cold turkey' and suddenly stop consuming caffeine, it is wise to plan this change. It makes sense that any possible withdrawal symptoms are timed so that they don't coincide with days when its important for you to be feeling your best. The good news is that any withdrawal symptoms are usually completely cleared after five to seven days when you should be feeling very much better.

You may decide it will be easier for you to cut down gradually, just as you would wean yourself from any other powerful drug. This should reduce the severity of any withdrawal symptoms you experience. This approach makes the withdrawal a longer process which can be frustrating if you are impatient to see what you feel like when you are completely caffeine-free. The withdrawal from caffeine will not be completed until after you have totally eliminated all the caffeine from your diet.

If symptoms get too bad then you can try the 'hair of the dog' method and take a few sips of your preferred source of caffeine – just enough to take the edge off a headache.

Coping with the unpleasant withdrawal symptoms such as headaches can be made easier by drinking plenty of water to help with the detoxification process. A minimum of eight glasses throughout the day is recommended. If symptoms get too bad then you can try the 'hair of the dog' method and take a few sips of your preferred source of caffeine – just enough to take the edge off a headache. To help with coffee cravings during this time you could try reducing the amount of alcohol, meat, sugar, flour, grains and salt in your diet, all of which tend to increase the desire for caffeine, and coffee in particular.

Caffeine Alternatives and Substitutes Survey

Making changes to the amount of caffeine you consume means that you will need to find some alternative drinks and foods to substitute instead. In the following table you will find a list of some grain drinks that can be used in place of coffee and also some alternatives for traditional tea. You need to consider these grain-based 'coffee alternatives' and herbal teas more as drinks that you can have in place of coffee or tea rather than drinks that are meant to taste exactly the same. There are many you can choose between and the taste of these caffeine-free 'alternatives' does vary between different brands, so keep trying until you find those you like.

If the cost of experimenting with new foods and the risk of buying a jar or packet that you don't like and then won't use is cause for concern, then you could consider the idea of arranging a tasting session with friends. This is a fun way for you to share the cost, and also the risk, of buying something you may find you don't like. If you select a variety of brands with a range of different ingredients then each person in the group will probably find something to take home that they like.

Caffeine-free Alternatives to Coffee, Tea and Chocolate

Caffeine-free Coffee 'Alternatives'

These are made from various grains, including rye and barley, plus chicory, figs and even acorns! They all taste different so keep sampling them until you find the one you like.

Ingredients	Barley Cup	Bambu	Caro	Chicory	Dandelion root	Dandelion coffee	Nocaf	Wake Up	Yannoh
Barley	✓		✓				✓	✓	✓
Malted barley			✓						✓
Chicory	✓	✓	✓	✓			✓	✓	✓
Rye	✓	✓	✓				✓	✓	✓
Figs		✓					✓	✓	
Wheat		✓							
Acorns		✓							✓
Chickpeas							✓	✓	
Dandelion root					✓	✓			
Lactose					✓				
Guarana								✓	

(Table header: **Brand name**)

Caffeine-free Tea 'Alternatives'

The word tea refers to the infusion process by which the drink is made, although we usually think of tea as meaning the traditional 'cuppa' made from black tea leaves. There are many alternative teas that can be brewed either from the loose herb or from 'bags'. Here are some that you could try.

CATS CLAW

This is a stimulating South American herb with many therapeutic properties.

ROOIBOSH (RED BUSH) TEA

This closely resembles 'real' tea but is naturally caffeine free, although it does contain tannin.

HERBAL TEAS

These are usually sold as the individual herb and are all known for their therapeutic properties, e.g. Camomile, Echinacea, Fennel, Peppermint, Nettle, St John's Wort.

HERBAL TEA MIXTURES

These are often mixtures of herbs and spices, specially formulated to have either a stimulating or a relaxing effect, e.g. Yogi Tea, Mu tea

FRUITY HERBAL TEAS

These may be sold individually but are usually sold as blends, often with colourful names and packaging, e.g. Apple, Blackcurrant, Cherry, Raspberry, Strawberry.

Caffeine-free Chocolate 'Alternatives'

The closest-tasting food to chocolate, that is not chocolate, is carob. It is sold as bars, used in sweets, spreads and can be bought, often in powder form, for milk shakes, hot drinks or baking. Carob is made from the carob bean and does not contain caffeine.

Nut butters such as almond nut butter (which is simply roasted and ground almonds) share the sweet taste and creamy texture that makes chocolate so appealing. They contain valuable nutrients and beneficial polyunsatured essential fats. Nut butters can be used to make alternative snacks to chocolate by spreading it on to oatcakes, rice cakes or other crackers. For a real treat, try dipping fruit such as cherries into almond nut butter.

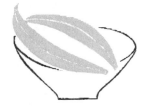

8

Emotional Roller-coaster Rides

Highs and lows in mood and energy can be linked to highs and lows in blood sugar levels.

Highs and lows in mood and energy can be linked to highs and lows in blood sugar levels. Blood sugar is affected by the food we eat and drink, particularly sweet, sugary and starchy foods. We may eat these foods because we enjoy the taste or need the high of almost instant energy they provide. Unfortunately, these highs can be followed by lows in mood and energy that are not so pleasant. Rescuing ourselves, perhaps by eating another starchy or sugary snack or by having a stimulant-containing drink, often seems to be the only option. In this way our days can become a never-ending emotional roller-coaster ride.

This chapter looks at the highs and lows of emotions and energy and the changes in blood sugar levels that can be related to what you are eating. There is a menu of tried-and-tested methods to enable you to successfully manage these fluctuating blood sugar levels. You will discover how you can manipulate your diet to manage your moods and so regain an emotional equilibrium. You will be able to take greater control of how you feel simply by changing what, and when, you eat.

Before looking in detail at what you are eating (and what may need to change), you may like to try the next exercise: 'A Day in the Life of You'. This allows you to chart your highs and lows over a 24-hour period. It will illustrate how much of a problem you may have with fluctuating moods and energy. Then, by reading through this chapter, you will discover what the highs and lows in your chart mean and – if change is needed – the best way for you to start.

A Day in the Life of You

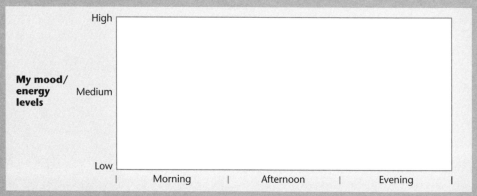

Fig 21 – Blood sugar/mood chart

You can do this exercise by reflecting on what is typical for you in terms of changes in mood and energy levels over a 24-hour period.

- Start by copying the chart above onto a piece of paper.
- Throughout the day (or when you look back at the end of the day) trace a line on the chart that shows how high and how low your moods and energy levels rise and fall.
- Add to the line marks to show when you eat a main meal, when you have snacks and also when you have hot, cold or alcoholic drinks.
- To complete the picture you could also show (e.g. in a different colour) when you smoke or take any medication that affects your mood or energy.

Now, if your chart looks rather like a roller-coaster ride, then the information in this chapter is going to be particularly useful for you. Please continue reading to find out how you could change a Mood and Energy Levels chart that looks like a 'mountain range' to one that shows a more calm and gentle passage through the day.

Of course, treating mood and energy levels as being closely related may be over-simplifying how you feel. There may be times when you know rest is more appropriate for you but, for a number of reasons, you 'keep going'. Sometimes it is anxiety that drives us to 'keep busy'. Perhaps we feel the need to distract ourselves from difficult feelings or do something to avoid experiencing certain emotions. The process of becoming more aware of our moods and being able to 'read' our real energy levels more accurately can help us to make better decisions about what we really need to be doing at different times.

Secret Sugar

The average person consumes roughly 20 teaspoons of added sugar every day.

If you consider yourself to be the 'average person' then, according to statistics, you could be eating the equivalent of 100g (which is roughly 20 teaspoons) of added sugar every day. As average figures are just guides to what is commonplace, you could be eating much more than this amount. Nearly half of us add table sugar (sucrose) to coffee or tea or sprinkle it on our breakfast cereals. But most of the sugars we eat are hidden in processed foods, put there by the manufacturers who wish to cater for our sweet tooth, our need for convenience and foods with a longer shelf-life. A can of cola drink may contain about 35g of sugar – equivalent to about seven teaspoons of white table sugar. A tin of baked beans can contain almost 25g of added sugar – equivalent to five teaspoons! And then, of course, there are sweets, biscuits and cakes which almost always contain added sugar…

To give you an idea of the hidden sugar in foods, here are some everyday sugar-containing foods listed with the amount of sugar they contain per 100g of food. You can read the amounts given 'per 100g' as a percentage if this is easier to imagine. You can also think of 5g sugar as being equivalent to about one teaspoon of table sugar.

Secret Sugar

	amount of sugar per 100g	approx % sugar content	equivalent no. of teaspoons table sugar
malted milk bedtime drink	47g	47%	9
chocolate breakfast cereal	39g	39%	8
crunchy cornflake breakfast cereal	34g	34%	7
plain chocolate biscuits	32.4g	33%	6
tin custard	11.9g	12%	2.5
tinned sweet corn	6.5g	6.5%	1.5
baked beans	6g	6%	1
strawberry yoghurt	5.6g	5%	1
tin chicken sauce	5.6g	5%	1
tomato soup	5.3g	5%	1

It is worth periodically checking the labels of your favourite brands to keep an eye on what exactly you are eating.

You can find this information for yourself by reading the food manufacturers' labels (there are some guidelines for how to read food labels later in this chapter). It is worth remembering that the ingredients of the same brand of prepared food can change – such as in response to consumer concerns about what is healthy. Recent examples include concerns over the level of salt in foods and whether the ingredients contain genetically modified foods. It is worth periodically checking the labels of your favourite brands to keep an eye on what exactly you are eating.

Sugar Checklist

Let's have a closer look at what you might be eating that contains added sugar. The list below shows some commonly eaten foods that often contain hidden added sugars. To be certain they contain sugar you will need to read the food label but if they taste sweet, the chances are they contain added sugar in some shape or form *(see the section on reading labels for help with this).* Don't be fooled by sweet-tasting 'no added sugar' foods as these probably contain artificial sweeteners instead. Artificial sweeteners are synthetic chemicals which may have a detrimental effect on the body with continuous long-term use. So, which of the foods below do you have more than once each week?

♣ Alcoholic drinks and mixers	♣ Frozen food
♣ Baked beans	♣ Fruit drinks
♣ Biscuits	♣ Honey
♣ Bread	♣ Hot chocolate drink
♣ Breakfast cereals	♣ Ice cream
♣ Buns	♣ Jam
♣ Cakes	♣ Ketchup
♣ Chocolate	♣ Malt
♣ Chutney and pickles	♣ Malted milk
♣ Cocoa	♣ Marmalade
♣ Condensed milk	♣ Mayonnaise
♣ Custard	♣ Milk shakes
♣ Evaporated milk	♣ Molasses
♣ Fizzy drinks	♣ Ovaltine

- ♣ Packet foods
- ♣ Pastries
- ♣ Peanut butter
- ♣ Pies
- ♣ Processed cheese
- ♣ Puddings
- ♣ Ready meals
- ♣ Relishes
- ♣ Rolls
- ♣ Sauces

- ♣ Soup
- ♣ Sweets
- ♣ Syrup
- ♣ Treacle
- ♣ Soft drinks and squash
- ♣ Table sugar
- ♣ Tinned foods
- ♣ Whipped cream
- ♣ Yoghurt

Sugar Blues

So what's wrong with sugar? The brain certainly needs fuel to function and its main energy source is sugar in the form of glucose. Glucose is obtained from the food we eat through the process of digestion which breaks down starches and sugars into glucose. Glucose passes into the bloodstream and is transported, in the form of 'blood glucose' or 'blood sugar', around the body as fuel to be used for energy.

The body is able to store glucose in the form of glycogen. This is kept in muscle tissue and in the liver and is readily available should it be needed. Excess sugar in the blood can also be converted into fat. This is the body's way of storing fuel for the longer-term, originally evolved to be a source of energy in times of hardship or famine.

Brain cells use some five times more glucose than other cells in the body and are very sensitive to changes in blood glucose levels. Low levels of blood glucose can produce aggression, anxiety, confusion, depression, fatigue and irritability, while levels that are too high also affect the normal functioning of the brain and can eventually result in a loss of consciousness. So, as always, it is a question of getting the balance right in order to feel good.

Blood glucose levels are related to what we eat. Both starches and sugars in food are types of carbohydrate. The carbohydrates we eat originally come from plant-based foods and are grouped and named according to how simple or complex they are in shape and size. Some of the different types of carbohydrates and some foods they come from are shown in the table below.

Carbohydrates in Foods

Sugars (Simple Carbohydrates)
Single sugars (monosaccharides)

Fructose   found in fruit, some vegetables and honey

Glucose   found in fruit, some vegetables and honey

Galactose   does not occur on its own in food

Double sugars (disaccharides)

Some single sugars can be paired up to form double sugars. The following all include glucose:

Glucose + Glucose = Maltose   found in sprouting grains such as barley

Glucose + Fructose = Sucrose (i.e. table sugar)   found in sugar cane or sugar beet

Glucose + Galactose = Lactose   'milk sugar' found in milk and milk products

Starches (Complex Carbohydrates)
Polysaccharides

Amylopectin   e.g. found in wheat, corn

Amylose   e.g. found in barley, rye, quinoa

Eating too many refined starchy or sugar-rich foods will affect your mood and mental functioning for the worse.

If the Mood and Energy Levels chart you completed earlier shows an emotional roller-coaster ride, then the type of carbohydrates you are eating could be the culprit. Eating too many refined starchy or sugar-rich foods will affect your mood and mental functioning for the worse. This effect will be exaggerated if you are someone who is particularly sensitive to the carbohydrates in food. The following exercise is in the form of a quiz that will show if sugar sensitivity is likely to be a problem for you.

Am I Sugar Sensitive?

Listed below are some symptoms that suggest a sensitivity to the carbohydrates in food. The more answers you tick, the more likely you are to be 'sugar sensitive'.

- I often feel dizzy, shaky, faint, fuzzy-headed or have difficulty concentrating
- I usually feel drowsy or tired during the day
- I get headaches quite often
- I sweat a lot during the night or day
- I am often anxious, fearful or depressed
- I get moody or irritable, angry or feel aggressive unexpectedly
- I get stressed out easily
- I tend to put on weight easily
- I tend to graze on food throughout the day
- I often feel I need a tea, coffee, cola, cigarette or alcoholic drink
- I've got a sweet tooth – I like eating sweet things
- I really like eating bread, cereal, pasta

The more of these statements that apply to you, the more likely it is that a sensitivity to carbohydrates is what's behind the highs and lows in your mood and energy. Fortunately, there are established ways of managing your body's response to carbohydrates so that you can still eat starchy and sweet-tasting foods yet avoid an emotional roller-coaster ride.

But you may be wondering how you came to be like this in the first place. The answer is likely to be a combination of a genetic predisposition that you inherited from your parents, together with environmental factors that include a lifestyle where you often skip meals, use a large amount of stimulants (such as caffeine in coffee just to 'keep you going'), and eat a diet high in starchy or sugary foods and snacks. Sudden or major life-changes or illnesses can also initiate a shift in the normally-functioning balance mechanisms of the body.

Let us now look more closely at what can be happening in the body of a sugar-sensitive person.

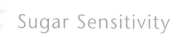

Sugar Sensitivity

Compare your 'Day in the Life of You' chart (which you completed earlier) with the following two charts. The first is the chart of a sugar-sensitive person and the second – which shows less of a roller-coaster ride – is the chart of someone who has their blood sugar level response to foods (and the associated highs and lows in mood and energy) much more under control.

Blood sugar level

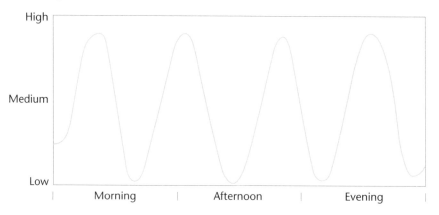

Fig 22 – Chart of a sugar-sensitive person

The bodies of sugar-sensitive people tend to have a stronger reaction to eating sugary foods. For these people, the normal increase in blood sugar (which occurs within an hour of eating) can be higher and more rapid than for non-sugar-sensitive people. What happens next is that the pancreas produces insulin to get the blood sugar level down again but tends to overcompensate, producing too much insulin which sends the blood sugar down to a level which is now too low. Symptoms of hypoglycaemia or 'low blood sugar' (which can occur about one to four hours after eating) include aggression, anxiety, confusion, depression, fatigue and irritability.

When blood sugar levels are too low we have a situation where a hit of sugar is needed quickly. But the sugar-sensitive person who eats a fast energy-releasing food then repeats the rapid rise in blood sugar level which is followed once more by the steep drop in blood sugar some hours later. Such a roller-coaster ride in blood sugar level usually results in similar highs and lows of mood and energy.

Blood sugar level

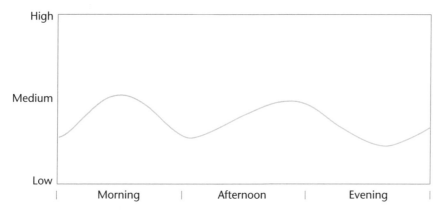

Fig 23 – Chart when blood sugar levels are under control

The blood sugar curve of a sugar-sensitive person who eats to avoid the highs and lows has no extreme peaks or troughs. The chart rises gently in response to eating something and falls slowly as the sugar is used for energy or stored. Blood sugar levels are fairly stable and predictable.

The Glycaemic Index

The Glycaemic Index (GI) is a relatively new way of measuring the effect that a food has on blood glucose levels. If you eat pure glucose it can be absorbed undigested into the bloodstream to produce the maximum response on blood glucose levels in the shortest time. In the making of the index, glucose is usually chosen to represent the maximum possible score a food can have – an index rating of 100. Scores in the Index range from 0 to 100. Foods with a lower GI score do not raise blood sugar levels as much as foods with a higher score. Therefore, when using the GI to decide what to eat, it is recommended to choose those foods with a low Glycaemic Index.

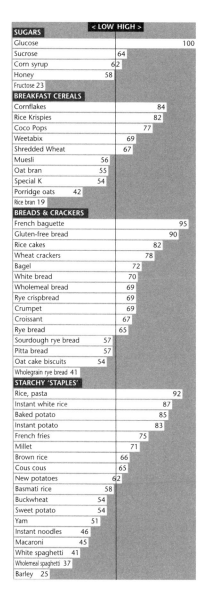

SUGARS	< LOW HIGH >
Glucose	100
Sucrose	64
Corn syrup	62
Honey	58
Fructose	23

BREAKFAST CEREALS	
Cornflakes	84
Rice Krispies	82
Coco Pops	77
Weetabix	69
Shredded Wheat	67
Muesli	56
Oat bran	55
Special K	54
Porridge oats	42
Rice bran	19

BREADS & CRACKERS	
French baguette	95
Gluten-free bread	90
Rice cakes	82
Wheat crackers	78
Bagel	72
White bread	70
Wholemeal bread	69
Rye crispbread	69
Crumpet	69
Croissant	67
Rye bread	65
Sourdough rye bread	57
Pitta bread	57
Oat cake biscuits	54
Wholegrain rye bread	41

STARCHY 'STAPLES'	
Rice, pasta	92
Instant white rice	87
Baked potato	85
Instant potato	83
French fries	75
Millet	71
Brown rice	66
Cous cous	65
New potatoes	62
Basmati rice	58
Buckwheat	54
Sweet potato	54
Yam	51
Instant noodles	46
Macaroni	45
White spaghetti	41
Wholemeal spaghetti	37
Barley	25

SNACKS/DRINKS	< LOW HIGH >
Corn crisps	72
Mars Bar	68
Muesli bar	61
Popcorn	55
Potato crisps	54
Grapefruit juice	48
Orange Juice	46
Apple juice	40

FRUIT	
Watermelon	72
Breadfruit	68
Pineapple	66
Cantaloupe melon	65
Raisin	64
Apricot	57
Sultana	56
Mango	55
Banana	55
Paw Paw	54
Kiwi fruit	52
Grape	46
Orange	44
Peach	42
Plum	39
Pear	38
Apple	38
Apricot (dried)	31
Grapefruit	25
Cherry	22

VEGETABLES	
Parsnips	97
Swede	72
Beetroot	64
Sweetcorn	55
Carrots	49
Peas (frozen)	48
Tomato soup	33

LEGUMES	
Baked beans	48
Black-eyed beans	41
Pinto beans	39
Haricot beans	38
Chickpeas	33
Yellow split peas	32
Butter beans	31
Kidney beans	29
Red lentils	25
Soya beans	18

Fig 24 – The Glycaemic Index of Foods

Foods are still being tested for their Glycaemic Index value and the list above gives the currently available GI values for some more common foods.

The GI of a food shows the effect that food has on blood sugar levels when it is compared to pure glucose, which has been given the maximum score of 100.

Foods with a lower GI score do not raise blood sugar levels as much as foods with a higher score and are therefore a better choice for avoiding the extreme highs (and the subsequent lows) associated with fluctuating blood sugar levels.

Using the GI

When a food with a high GI score is combined with a food with low GI score (in approximately equal amounts) the result is a meal that has a medium GI score: HIGH GI FOOD + LOW GI FOOD = MEDIUM GI MEAL. So, as you probably can't eat only low GI foods, as long as the mixture of foods in your meal contains some foods with a low GI, the combined effect will be a medium GI meal that should not result in a sharp rise in blood sugar levels.

A lower GI score is usually explained by the slow rate at which that food is digested. In other words, slowly-digested foods tend to have a lower GI and the index can be seen as a measure of the speed at which the sugars in food are released into the bloodstream.

There are several factors which can slow down the rate of digestion. These include the amount of fibre, the amount of fat, the amount of protein and the type of starch.

- The presence of whole fibre lowers the GI of a food. For example, a whole grapefruit has a GI of only 25 but grapefruit juice, which contains little fibre, scores a much higher 48. Similarly, wholegrain rye bread is a low 41 but ordinary rye bread is a high-scoring 65.
- Potatoes are generally high, having a score above 60, but add some fat and the GI comes down. So a plain potato will have a higher GI than potatoes served with fat such as butter or olive oil. It also seems that eating potatoes with their skins on (containing fibre) will lower the GI of the potato meal.
- Foods such as peas, beans and lentils, because of their protein content, have a low GI, all scoring under 60.
- Starch in food comes in different shapes and sizes. The type of starch in food affects its GI score because of how easily it is unravelled and digested by the body. It seems to be the case that the more amylose starch a food contains, the lower the GI score. Foods with a relatively high amylopectin starch content have higher GI values. For example, wheat and corn are high in amylopectin, which makes them a relatively fast-releasing food and gives them higher GI scores. Barley, rye and quinoa, on the other hand, contain higher amounts of amylose starch, which makes them slower-releasing foods, and so they score lower on the index. Generally speaking, rice has a high GI score due to its high amylopectin content. However, basmati rice has more amylose and is therefore slower-releasing and so would be the rice of choice for creating a low GI meal.

As a general rule, sugars tend to score high on the GI. The exception to this rule is fructose which is commonly known as 'fruit sugar'. This has a GI score of only 23. Fructose is available in health food stores as a substitute for table sugar and is often sold as a product for people with diabetes. The GI of honey depends on the blend of sugars it contains and how much fructose is present in the mix. Apple juice is often recommended as an alternative sweetener because it generally has a relatively high fructose content which lowers its GI.

Buckwheat and Lentils

Type: Dinner
Equipment: 2 medium pans, hob
Preparation time: 5 mins
Cooking time: 25 mins

The benefits of buckwheat, including its low Glycaemic Index, are explained in the recipe for Sweet Potato Cakes (*page 16*). Lentils also have a low GI so, in combination with the buckwheat, this makes a slow energy-releasing meal that will keep you going for much longer. Lentils cook quickly, compared to other legumes, and are also a vegetarian source of tryptophan protein which is then converted in the brain to the good mood neurotransmitter serotonin. The toasted pumpkin and sesame seeds are more than just a texture-adding garnish, as they contain essential fats and good mood minerals including zinc. Vegetable stock that is gluten/dairy/yeast-free can be purchased from health-food stores.

Ingredients (per person)

1 tbsp olive oil
30g/1oz/¼ cup chopped fresh onion
1 garlic clove, chopped/crushed
1–2 sticks celery, chopped finely
100g/4oz/1 cup red split lentils
1 litre/2 pints/4 cups vegetable stock
100g/4oz/1 cup buckwheat groats
handful each of sunflower and pumpkin seeds

Method

1   Gently sauté the onion, garlic and celery in the olive oil.
2   Rinse the lentils and add to the pan with half of the vegetable stock.
3   Cover and simmer gently, adding more water if it runs dry, until lentils are soft and blended together (about 25 mins).
4   Meanwhile, in a separate pan, cook the buckwheat. To bring out the nutty flavour of buckwheat, dry toast the groats until lightly browned. Carefully (because of the steam) add the remaining vegetable stock. Cover and simmer gently, adding more water if it runs dry until groats are tender (about 20 mins).
5   Serve sprinkled with pumpkin and sunflower seeds.
6   This dish can be enjoyed as it is but also goes well with a crunchy green salad.

Ready?	Until you are experienced enough to recognize what lentils and buckwheat look like when cooked, you will probably need to taste them to be certain.
Underdone	Lentils and buckwheat still crunchy to taste.
Just right	Buckwheat just slightly firm. Lentils soft and blended together.
Overdone	Buckwheat groats becoming soggy and beginning to look like a porridge mixture. Lentils soft and blended together but now drying out and sticking to the pan.
Trouble-shooting tip	If you have overcooked the buckwheat and/or lentils they'll still taste good but just won't look as appealing. It's easy to do a rescue job by combining the buckwheat and lentils and pressing the mixture firmly into a bread tin or small oven-proof dish. This can then be cooked in a medium oven (180°C/350°F/Gas Mark 4) to emerge about 20 mins later as a lentil and buckwheat 'bake'.

Ten Ways to Improve Sugar-sensitivity

If you think you might be sugar-sensitive and would like to level out the highs and lows of energy and mood to experience life on a more even keel, there are several changes you could make to achieve this which can be effective within weeks if not days. The more of these changes you can manage, the more benefits you are likely to experience in the shortest time. All of the following recommendations can help and include the idea of the Glycaemic Index of foods explained above.

1. Cut Down on the Sugar You Add to Food

You have probably gathered that too much sugar, particularly the refined sort added to food, is not going to be good for your emotional and mental health, especially if eaten in large amounts on a daily basis. A reduction in the amount you are eating is likely to be needed. But a word of warning: sugar can be experienced as a highly addictive substance.

Eating large amounts of sugar on a regular basis may create an addictive-type relationship with sugar that can be difficult to change.

Eating sugar-rich foods is thought to trigger the release of pleasure-giving brain chemicals called endorphins which 'reward' us for eating these foods. Eating large amounts of sugar on a regular basis may create an addictive-type relationship with sugar that can be difficult to change. We have no doubt evolved to find the taste of sugar extremely enjoyable because it guarantees an instant energy fix that in the past may have been essential for our survival. Sugar (mostly in the form of honey or sweet fruits) would have been harder for our cave-dwelling ancestors to obtain compared with the availability of sugar today. Concentrated sugar (for our ancestors) would have been an extremely valuable food compared with what is needed for the survival of modern man.

You may find that if you suddenly exclude all concentrated sugars from your diet you experience unpleasant withdrawal symptoms and feel worse before you feel better, as your body and brain adjust to the change. For this reason it is often easier if you reduce your sugar intake slowly and re-train your taste buds gradually. Your first step could be to cut down on the quantity of concentrated sugars in your daily diet. Start by reducing the amount of table sugar you add to tea or coffee and sprinkle over breakfast cereal, or indeed over any other foods you eat. Try setting yourself the target to re-educate your taste buds to enjoy less sugar within a few weeks or months – whatever feels comfortable to you.

SETTING TARGETS

In setting goals, begin by making a note of the specific change you want to make. If you wish to cut down on a food such as sugar, start by noting how much you are having now. Next, decide on a realistic timescale to work with. This may be a week, it could be a month. Choose whatever feels comfortable for you, but try and get the balance right between making it too difficult for yourself and too easy a target. Then break down the bigger change you want to make into smaller 'mini-targets'. You will need to reach each of these in turn if you are to be successful in achieving your overall goal.

For example, John habitually added two teaspoons of white table sugar to tea and drank five to six cups per day, a daily total of 10–12 teaspoons (or approximately 50–60g sugar) consumed this way. At first he decided not to change the amount of sugar in the first cup of the day as this was the drink most important to him. He would, however, attempt to cut down on the amount he was adding to his cuppas later on in the day. John set himself the target of reducing the amount of sugar in his tea by half a teaspoon per cup per week so that by the fourth week he would be drinking his tea without sugar. After the second week, the first cup of the day which contained his habitual two teaspoons was now tasting too sweet. John continued to reduce the amount he was using and was able to reach his goal of drinking tea without sugar one month later. He said it even tasted good this way and if someone forgot and made him a cup of tea with two sugars in he found it 'horribly sweet'.

LOOKING AT LABELS

To find out the sugar content of tinned, packet and frozen foods you will need to become a food detective and start to read the labels. Here are some tips to help you decode the information provided by the manufacturers.

- Ingredients are listed in descending order of quantity. Sugar found listed near the beginning means that the food has a high amount of sugar compared to the other ingredients.
- Be wary of 'no added sugar' as this can mean just 'no added sucrose' and other types of sugar may have been added instead.
- In order to make the recognizable sugar content appear low, manufacturers may list the sugars they have used in their different forms, but they all have a similar effect on the body. *(See the table 'Sugar By Any Other Name', below for a list of other words that mean 'sugar'.)* Quick tip: any words ending in 'ose' such as glucose, sucrose, maltose, dextrose, will be describing sugars.

♣   Foods that don't contain sugar often contain fruit juice instead. Foods sweetened with apple juice usually make the better choice *(for the reason why, read the section on the Glycaemic Index of foods, above)*.

♣   'Diet' or 'low-sugar' foods also contain artificial sweeteners such as Acesulfame-K, Aspartame (e.g. Nutrasweet, Canderel), Saccharin and Thaumatin. These are synthetic chemicals which may have a detrimental effect on the body with continuous long-term use.

♣   The 'nutritional information' section of food labels is particularly useful. In it you can find the amount of carbohydrate present, usually listed 'per 100g' of that food and sometimes also as the amount 'per serving'. The carbohydrate content may then be further divided into the amount of starch and the amount of sugar. It is generally better to have carbohydrates in the form of starch rather than sugar, so look out for the amount of sugar that's listed.

1. Food name: there is a subtle but important difference between raspberry yoghurt and raspberry flavour yoghurt (which may not contain any real raspberries at all).

8. Under the amount of carbohydrates in the food may also be shown the amount of starch and/or sugar present.

9. Under the amount of fat in the food may also be shown the amount of saturated, monounsaturated and/or polyunsaturated fats present.

6. The big e means that on average the quantity should be accurate although there may be slight variations between the weight of each pack.

2. Ingredients are listed in descending order of weight.

7. This shows the energy value of 100g of the food measured in kilocalories or kilojoules.

10. Sodium is a component of table salt (sodium chloride). To work out the equivalent amount of table salt, multiply the sodium content by 2.5. One teaspoon of table salt weighs approximately 3g.

3. Storage instructions, if appropriate, should be provided.

4. A 'best before' or 'sell by' date needs to be included.

5. Name and address of manufacturer or seller must be given.

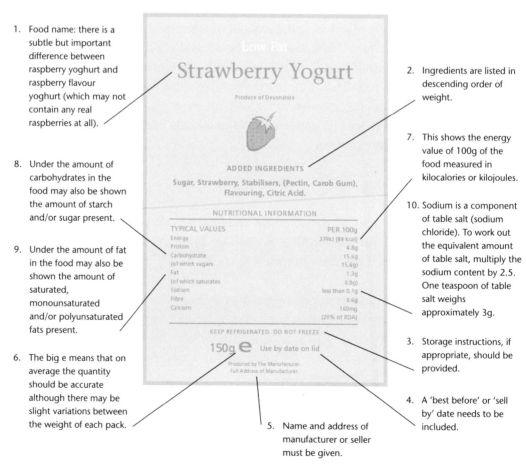

Fig 25 – Food label illustration

Sugar by Any Other Name...

Acesulfame-K (E950): An artificial chemical sweetener.

Alitame: An artificial chemical sweetener.

Amazake: A sweet purée containing simple sugars glucose and fructose formed by fermenting rice or millet.

Aspartame (E951): An artificial chemical sweetener.

Barbados sugar: A dark, moist, partly refined sugar. Also called Muscovado.

Barley syrup: Usually called malt syrup, containing mostly maltose. Made by fermenting cooked barley and then straining and heating to form a sticky syrup.

Black treacle: Another name for molasses.

Brown sugar: Refined soft sucrose crystals coated in molasses syrup.

Burnt sugar: Another name for caramel.

Canderel: The trade name for the artificial sweetener aspartame.

Caramel: Burnt sugar or syrup (used for colouring spirits).

Corn syrup: Produced from cornstarch and containing fructose and glucose/dextrose.

Cyclamates (E952): An artificial chemical sweetener.

Date sugar: Sugar made from dates.

Demerara: Can be white sugar dyed with caramel.

Dextrose: Another name for glucose. Also called corn sugar. Dextrose from corn is often blended with sucrose to make refined table sugar.

Fructose: Naturally occurring fruit sugar used in the same way as sucrose (table sugar).

Golden syrup: A by-product of sugar-cane or sugar-beet refining.

Glucose/Glucose Syrup: A naturally occurring sugar usually manufactured from maize (sweet corn).

Honey: a natural combination of glucose, fructose, maltose and sucrose. May contain added sugar.

Isomalt (E953): A mixture of sugar 'alcohols' which can be naturally occurring in fruit but also commercially produced.

Lactitol (E966): A sugar 'alcohol' which can be naturally occurring in fruit but is also commercially produced from other plant sources.

Lactose and Lactate: Sugars derived from milk.

L(a)evulose: Another name for the fruit sugar fructose.

Malitol/Malitol syrup (E965): A sugar 'alcohol' which can be naturally occurring in fruit but is also commercially produced from other plant sources.

Malt syrup: Sometimes called barley syrup, containing mostly maltose.

Maltose: Found in sprouting grains such as barley.

Mannitol (Manna sugar) (E421): A sugar 'alcohol' which can be naturally occurring in fruit but is also commercially produced from other plant sources.

Maple syrup: The concentrated sap of 40+-year-old maple trees.

Molasses: Sometimes called black treacle, it is the strong-tasting residue left when cane sugar is refined.

Muscovado: A dark, moist, partly refined sugar. Sometimes called Barbados sugar.

Neotame: An artificial chemical sweetener.

Neohesperidine DC (E959): An artificial chemical sweetener.

Nutrasweet: A trade name for the artificial sweetener aspartame.

Raw sugar: Obtained from the evaporation of sugar cane juice.

Rice sugar: Sugar made from rice.

Saccharin (E954): An artificial chemical sweetener.

Sorbitol/Sorbitol syrup (E420): A sugar 'alcohol' which can be naturally occurring in fruit but is also commercially produced from other plant sources.

Sucralose: An artificial chemical sweetener.

Sucrose: Obtained by refining sugar beet and sugar cane which involves extraction of the juice, purification and concentration.

Stevia: A herb which can be used as a sweetener.

Table sugar: Another name for white sugar (sucrose).

Thaumatin (E957): An artificial chemical sweetener.

Total invert sugar: A liquid sweetener formed by splitting sucrose into glucose and fructose.

Turbinado: A refined 'raw' sugar with the impurities and molasses removed.

White sugar: Another name for sucrose.

Xylitol (E967): Sugar 'alcohols' which can be naturally occurring in fruit but also commercially produced from other plant sources.

'EMPTY' CALORIES

Refined sugars which have been added to food and drinks do not contain any other nutrients and are good for one thing only – calories or 'energy' so they are often referred to as 'empty'. Worse still, eating concentrated sugary foods also robs the body of essential minerals and vitamins. Every time these sugar-rich foods are consumed in excess, the body is thrown out of balance. In trying to get things back on a even keel, the body has to draw on supplies of minerals such as chromium and magnesium and B-vitamins, and these are valuable nutrients that are needed elsewhere in the body.

2. Cut Down on Free Sugars

The good news for sugar-lovers is that not all sugars are bad.

The good news for sugar-lovers is that not all sugars are bad. However, the effect on mental health does depend on what type of sugar you eat as well as how much. Natural sugars, such as those found in whole fruits and vegetables, tend to make much healthier choices. These sugars, called 'intrinsic' sugars because they are 'locked in' to the food, are not broken down by the process of digestion and released into the bloodstream as quickly as 'extrinsic' or free sugars. Intrinsic sugars have to be pressed, processed, cooked or digested before they are released. Consequently, there isn't such a sugar 'high' produced after eating them. Neither do they result in the drop in energy and mood that is often the price to pay an hour or so afterwards. Unfortunately, much of the sugar in the modern diet is the more harmful 'free' or 'extrinsic' sugars which are not so effectively 'locked' in to food.

Although fruit and vegetable juices do contain much goodness in the form of vitamins and minerals, if you are very sensitive to sugars in food you may benefit from reducing the amount of concentrated juices you drink. Fruits and vegetables that have been juiced no longer contain as much fibre as the whole food. The natural sugars that were originally locked in now have similar effects on the body as added sugar. Instead, you could reduce the sugar 'hit' you get from drinking concentrated juices by diluting them with water. This may be a change to take slowly as you re-train your sense of taste, but aim for a drink that is made up of at least half juice with the remainder as water.

3. Change from 'White' to 'Brown' Foods

Whole foods or 'brown' foods have many health benefits over refined or 'white' foods. If you eat wholefoods such as whole (rather than juiced) fruit and vegetables, these will automatically contain more nutrients which are beneficial for emotional and mental health. Wholefoods also contain more fibre and generally produce only gentle rises and falls in blood sugar levels.

Whole foods also include whole grains. To eat whole grains you will need to choose 'brown' or 'wholemeal' versions of foods such as wholemeal bread or wholemeal pasta. These foods won't have been made using refined or white flours. Brown rice is another good example: when rice is refined, the outer coating of the grain is removed (unfortunately taking much of the goodness with it) in order to leave 'white' rice. So in this context, brown is definitely better.

A 'quick fix' option that can help restore some nutrients and fibre to refined foods is to add bran such as oat or rice bran. Oat or rice brans are preferred as they are less likely to irritate the digestive system and can be added in baking or to foods such as breakfast cereals. But for the most part, increasing the amount of whole foods in your diet seems to make more sense than adding back the nutrients and fibre as bran.

The table below contains some examples of brown and white versions of common foods.

Replacing 'White' Foods with 'Brown'

white rice	brown rice
white bread	wholemeal bread
white pasta	wholemeal pasta
French baguette bread	wholemeal bap
pastries/cakes made with white flour	pastries/cakes made with wholemeal flour

4. Include Some Protein with Every Meal

Meals and snacks that contain protein will digest more slowly and as a result 'keep you going' for longer.

The effect that starchy or sugary foods have on blood sugar levels is reduced if it is accompanied by some protein. Meals and snacks that contain protein will digest more slowly and as a result 'keep you going' for longer. For example, the protein content of breakfast can be increased by adding nuts and seeds to cereal or spreading nut butter such as almond nut butter onto toast. Of course, the traditional cooked breakfast containing bacon and egg is a protein-rich meal but because of its saturated fat content, this is not recommended for every breakfast! Later on in the day, a handful of nuts or seeds or a cracker spread with nut or seed 'butters' can make a quick and tasty protein-containing snack.

Protein-containing Foods

- meat
- fish
- cheese
- eggs

- beans
- nuts
- seeds

5. Eat Breakfast

Breakfast is an important meal for establishing an even blood-sugar ride through the rest of the day.

When time is short it is tempting to skip breakfast. Many sugar-sensitive people don't feel like eating early in the morning, preferring just a cup of tea or coffee to start the day. Those concerned about their weight often think that by not eating breakfast it will help with their diet. All of these people, especially if they experience highs and lows in mood and energy throughout the day, can be doing themselves a disservice by skipping breakfast.

Each morning you are literally breaking an overnight fast when you eat breakfast. It is an important meal for establishing an even blood-sugar ride through the rest of the day. If breakfast contains food that releases its energy slowly, you could find that you can keep going until lunchtime, without a mid-morning slump and the need for a stimulant such as a coffee-and-doughnut boost (and the low that often follows). Examples of slow-releasing breakfasts include wholemeal toast with nut butter or fruit spread, oat-based muesli or a bowl of porridge.

As far as weight-gain is concerned, the more frequently blood sugar is raised, the more insulin is produced and more sugar is likely to be dumped as fat. High insulin levels also inhibit the body's breakdown of previously stored fat. So to avoid unnecessary weight gain, you need to avoid the highs (and lows) of fluctuating blood sugar levels.

6. Plan Meals Ahead

You know that you're going to have to eat at some point.

So often our good intentions are ruined for lack of planning. Waiting until you are really hungry and then finding that the only thing available to eat is a starchy, sugary snack can be a recipe for disaster. You will get the quick fix but, as we have seen, it may not last very long. Much better to invest some time earlier on to plan – even prepare – what you are going to eat later. You know that you're going to have to eat at some point so accept the fact that your body needs regular pit stops, and make sure you are equipped to fill up with the premium grade, slow-releasing type of fuel.

7. Eat at Regular Intervals and Eat Three Main Meals a Day

Eating at regular intervals is essential for managing sugar sensitivity. You will need to find out how frequently you need to eat in order to prevent your blood sugar levels dipping too low so that you start to feel unwell. If you are sugar sensitive it will certainly mean that you need to have at least three proper meals every day.

It could be that you need to eat something every couple of hours but what is important is to give yourself 'staging posts' throughout the day, at intervals which suit your metabolism. Once you have established what works for you in terms of which foods you need to eat and how often, and you have planned for these fuel stops, then you are free to forget about food and concentrate on other areas of your life for a time.

Having clearly-scheduled times when you stop and eat is also helpful for managing cravings or food 'addictions'. Once you have had your meal or snack you will know that, until the next scheduled food time, you don't really need to eat anything. You should find that it is helpful to have clearer boundaries between eating and not eating, rather than tending to 'pick' at food all day long.

8. Eat Snacks between Meals (and Before Bed) if Needed

Eating a slow-releasing carbohydrate food such as porridge or muesli or even a jacket potato an hour before bed can actually help you get to sleep and have a more comfortable night.

Eating at regular intervals for a sugar-sensitive person will probably mean eating snacks 'between meals'. Some people call this 'grazing' and it works as long as you choose slow energy-releasing foods. It also helps to have clear boundaries between eating and not-eating times (*see above*).

Eating last thing at night has long been thought to lead to a disturbed night's sleep. This could be true for you but the quality of your sleep may depend more on what you eat. It can be difficult to sleep on a full stomach but it is also hard to rest properly when blood sugar levels are low and your body is on the look-out for food. Eating a slow-releasing carbohydrate food such as porridge or muesli or even a jacket potato an hour before bed can actually help you get to sleep and have a more comfortable night.

Eating carbohydrates assists the process of absorbing tryptophan into the brain where it is converted into the brain chemical serotonin.

Eating carbohydrates before bed assists the process of absorbing tryptophan into the brain where it is converted into the brain chemical serotonin, which helps us to sleep. Choosing slow-releasing carbohydrates enables you to have this benefit without the disadvantages of the highs and lows produced by fast-releasing carbohydrates. *(See Chapters 2 and 3 for more information about carbohydrate cravings and the connection with tryptophan absorption and the brain chemical serotonin.)*

9. Be Prepared when Out and About

A bag of stop-gap snacks can smooth the way.

'Being prepared' is a useful mantra for the sugar-sensitive person to adopt. If you can make sure that you always have something with you to nibble on, you'll be able to avoid letting your blood sugar dip too low. And when you know you are kitted out with a selection of tasty snacks, you can feel more confident when out and about. Having to find something suitable to eat won't feel such a 'life-or-death' crisis if you have provisions in your bag. It can also provide you with more time so you can make better choices about where to go and what, where and when to eat a more substantial meal.

Carrying some emergency supplies with you is also a good idea even if you are going straight to a place where you know there will be food. Restaurant chefs, and home cooks as well, sometimes serve up their meals later than planned, and waiting for food can soon become difficult for the sugar-sensitive person. Also, you may find that what's on the menu isn't to your liking and you can't eat your fill. In this situation, a bag of stop-gap snacks can smooth the way. Portable snacks include popcorn, oatcakes, fruit, some raw vegetables, nuts, fruit and nut mix, seeds, flapjacks.

10. Cut Down on Stimulants

Cutting down on the amount of stimulants you have is crucial for improving emotional and mental health difficulties which are associated with fluctuating blood sugar levels. The main offenders are caffeine (found in coffee, tea, cola, chocolate) and nicotine in cigarettes. The use of nicotine is not covered in this handbook but caffeine is considered so important that it has been given a chapter (*Chapter 7*) of its own. In the meantime, you will find that your efforts to manage the amount and type of sugar in your diet will be even more effective when you can also reduce the stimulants you use.

Case Study: Mood Swings and PMS

Catherine, aged 36, often experienced mood swings, especially prior to menstruation. But they didn't cause concern and didn't interfere with her enjoyment of life. However, after a long-term relationship with her boyfriend broke down, she started to feel very low. Catherine was not sleeping very well and felt tired. She was increasingly miserable and was not eating properly – just snacks here and there. Catherine also craved sweet foods – particularly chocolate and cups of tea with sugar. Two weeks before her period her mood would plummet, and after three months of this she felt unable to cope with work.

Catherine's GP suggested that a low mood was normal after a relationship had ended and she was offered the antidepressant Prozac. Although Catherine agreed that feeling depressed following a break-up with a boyfriend was normal, she thought it strange she that she had such a low mood prior to her period rather than all the time. She therefore declined the medication and decided to seek help elsewhere.

She visited a nutritional therapist and was advised to follow a diet to improve her blood sugar control which would benefit her premenstrual syndrome (PMS) and mood swings. Catherine followed the advice she had been given and within two weeks was feeling 'completely different'. Her mood swings had disappeared and she was enjoying an increased feeling of emotional and mental wellbeing. Catherine now felt able to cope and even enjoy life once more. Six months later she was still reporting continuing success using the nutritional therapy approach to PMS and mood swings.

Alternative Sweeteners

Reducing the amount of sugar and re-educating your taste buds to enjoy the natural sweetness in foods is the ideal. But you may find there are some foods that you have to sweeten in order to enjoy them. So what are the healthier options?

Fructose: Naturally occurring 'fruit sugar' can be used in the same way as sucrose (table sugar). It is much sweeter than sucrose so about one-third less is needed. Commercially produced fructose is usually derived from corn so it may not suit those with a sensitivity to corn. It is suitable for diabetics as it does not require insulin for its assimilation and it has a very low Glycaemic Index. However, large amounts of fructose can raise the amount of triglycerides (fats) in the blood and it has the same effect as other sugars on gut dysbiosis such as candida overgrowth.

Fructo-oligosaccharides (FOS): A sweet-tasting type of indigestible fibre found in fruits and vegetables which can be used as a supplement to support the growth of beneficial bacteria in the gut. It does not raise blood sugar levels and can be added to drinks, cereals or yoghurt.

Fruit spreads: An alternative to jam or marmalade consisting of whole fruits and fruit juice and nothing else.

Fruit juice: Apple juice is often recommended as an alternative sweetener because it generally has a relatively high fructose and low glucose content. This means it will have less of an effect on raising blood sugar levels.

Honey: The blood sugar raising effect of honey depends on the blend of sugars it contains and how much fructose and glucose is present in the mix. Use sparingly and choose pure honey in order to avoid those brands that have had sugar added.

Stevia: A naturally sweet-tasting herb from the Aster food family. Suitable for diabetics. May have antibacterial qualities and can be used in cooking and baking as well as for drinks and to sweeten foods.

Supplement Your Sugar Cravings

The mineral most often found to help with sugar cravings is chromium.

Sugar metabolism requires that the minerals chromium and magnesium and the B-vitamins are available in the body. Large quantities of these nutrients are lost when foods are refined and the bran and germ of the grain, rich in nutrients, is removed. But eating whole foods such as whole grains – for example whole wheat found in wholemeal bread and pasta – can provide these essential nutrients. Symptoms due to imbalances in blood sugar levels should improve by making the changes described in this chapter but it may also help to include a daily nutritional supplement for a while.

The mineral most often found to help with sugar cravings is chromium. Chromium is found in foods such as mushrooms, whole grains and yeast. A chromium supplement taken in the form of chromium polynicotinate provides two major ingredients for making Glucose Tolerance Factor (GTF). These are organically bound chromium and niacin (nicotinic acid). GTF is the form in which chromium exerts its blood sugar controlling activity and many people have found that a GTF chromium supplement can help with their sugar cravings. The suggested dosage, and recommended maximum, is 200ug per day. Please note that chromium should not be given to diabetics taking insulin unless medically supervised.

Of course the body needs a wide range of nutrients to be healthy. So, if you can take a good-quality multimineral and vitamin supplement that contains chromium combined in a balanced formula with other nutrients, then so much the better. Better still, a consultation with a qualified nutritional therapist can provide an assessment of your nutrient levels and recommendations for a tailor-made supplement programme.

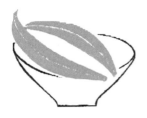

9

Good Mood Foods

The emphasis of this handbook is to support you in finding the foods that are right for your individual needs, preferences and lifestyle. You have been guided through a process of careful exploration of what you eat and drink. Having tried, tested and experienced first-hand the effects of changing your diet, you will have gained an insight into which foods are good for your emotional and mental health.

In this chapter you will find information on some good mood foods which you may find beneficial to include in your diet. Sensitivity to any food is possible so, if any of these recommended foods are a 'suspect' for you, please first check to see if they are suitable for you – perhaps by using the methods described in Chapter 5.

The Mind Meal for Mental Health

The Mind Meal aims to draw attention to the important relationship between food and mood.

The Mind Meal is one practical example of what can be done with some good mood foods. Launched by Mind (the mental health charity) in 2000, the Mind Meal aims to draw attention to the important relationship between food and mood. The recipes contain those foods generally recommended as being supportive for emotional and mental health. The simple, easy-to-prepare and tasty three-course meal provides an example of how these foods can be used. Mind continues to receive positive feedback from individuals and community groups who have tried and tested this menu of 'good mood foods'.

When you look at the list of ingredients, what the Mind Meal doesn't include is just as important as what it does contain. You won't, for example, find any artificial additives or added sugars. Neither does it provide any stimulants such as caffeine. The menu enables you to avoid wheat and milk – the two most common culprit foods associated with food sensitivities.

What the meal does provide are foods containing valuable vitamins, minerals and essential fats important for emotional and mental health. The oil-rich fish, as well as providing the vital omega-3 essential fats, is also a source of tryptophan. Tryptophan is the essential good mood protein-fragment which is also found in avocado, seeds, dried apricots and walnuts. Absorption of the tryptophan in the main course is assisted by the carbohydrates contained in the dessert. The tryptophan can be converted into the mood-enhancing brain chemical serotonin, and the banana and avocado also provide some ready-made serotonin. Because the meal has a medium-to-low Glycaemic Index, it will provide a slow release of energy that will keep you feeling good for longer.

The Mind Meal comprises the following three courses:

Wheat-free Pasta with Pesto and Oil-rich Fish
Avocado Salad & Seeds
Fruit & Oatcakes Dessert

- Serves two hungry people or up to four not-so-hungry people.
- Most of the ingredients will be available from your local food store. The ingredients marked * may be found in some general food stores but are almost certainly available at your local health-food store.
- Preparation time for the whole meal will be approximately 20 minutes, depending on how confident you are in the kitchen.

WHEAT-FREE PASTA WITH PESTO AND OIL-RICH FISH

250g/9oz (approx.) packet wheat-free pasta such as corn and vegetable pasta shells*
100g/4oz (approx.) pesto sauce (This is made from basil, olive oil, garlic, pine kernels and Parmesan cheese. If you can obtain vegan pesto* it will be dairy-free.)
170g/6oz (approx.) tin salmon or other oil-rich fish (e.g. mackerel, herring, sardines, pilchards) in brine, oil or spring water

1   Cook the pasta in boiling water as per the instructions on the packet.
2   When the pasta is ready, drain and transfer to a warmed serving dish. Add approx. 1 tablespoon pesto sauce per person and gently mix in with the pasta.
3   Open the tin of fish, drain liquid, remove or crush any large bones and flake with a fork. Add to serving dish containing pasta and pesto, and mix gently together.

Note: Tinned tuna is not a particularly good source of omega-3 oils as the canning process reduces the tuna's fat content. Fresh tuna makes a better choice.

AVOCADO SALAD & SEEDS

250g/8oz (approx.) bag mixed lettuce or 80g/4oz (approx.) bag watercress
1 avocado
a handful (approx. 25g/1oz/¹/4 cup) sunflower seeds
a handful (approx. 25g/1oz/¹/4 cup) pumpkin seeds*

1   Place the mixed salad in a serving dish.
2   Remove skin and stone from avocado. Cut avocado into small pieces and add to
    mixed salad.
3   Sprinkle on the seeds.
4   Serve plain, with olive oil or the salad dressing of your choice.

FRUIT & OATCAKES DESSERT

2 bananas
2 apples
8 dried apricots (preferably additive-free)
8–12 oatcakes
40g/2oz/¹/2 cup (broken) walnuts

1   Peel the bananas and rinse the apples and dried apricots.
2   Cut the fruit into small pieces (remove apple core) and place together in a small
    saucepan.
3   Add a minimum of 3 tablespoons of water and simmer gently for approx. 10 minutes or
    until fruit is soft, adding more water to prevent the mixture becoming too dry and
    sticking to the pan. (This tastes great as it is but, if available, you could add a dash of
    lemon juice and/or a teaspoon of chopped ginger and/or a pinch of cinnamon
    powder, according to your taste.)
4   Meanwhile arrange oatcakes in the bottom of individual bowls (you may have to break
    them into pieces to make them fit).
5   When fruit mixture is soft, pour into individual bowls to cover the oatcakes. If the fruit
    mixture contains enough liquid, the juices will soak into, and soften, the oatcakes.
6   Serve with a sprinkling of broken walnuts.

Good Mood Nutrients

Taking some nutritional supplements may be the only way to obtain what is needed to feel well.

To attribute how we think and feel as being entirely due to the effect of specific nutrients would obviously ignore the wide range of influences that affect emotional and mental health. Yet much of the (often confusing and contradictory) nutritional advice in the media arises from scientific research which has been conducted by focusing on individual nutrients and testing them to learn their specific effects in particular situations. The scientific testing of individual nutrients may not always reflect how the whole mind-and-body responds to food or functions in everyday circumstances outside of the laboratory. Further, this process tends to highlight certain individual nutrients which then become better known for their beneficial effects, whilst giving less attention to other nutrients which may be just as important.

All nutrients function together in an extremely complex network of supportive and antagonistic relationships. It is likely that the nutrients most compatible with the human mind-and-body are those found in food, rather than the substances that can be obtained from nutritional supplements. Although not all foods in nature are harmless to humans, our bodies have evolved over millions of years because we have been able to adapt to what we experience in our environment. Whole foods (rather than refined or overly processed products) which have been grown with the minimum artificial fertilizers, pesticides and herbicides, are going to be closest to what the human body is designed to deal with.

Yet, because the amount of nutrients within foods varies enormously, and the soil on which food is grown can be lacking in minerals, taking some nutritional supplements may be the only way to obtain what is needed to feel well.

A Matter of Fats

Fats matter a lot to emotional and mental health, with low levels in the diet being associated with symptoms that range from anxiety and depression to hyperactivity and schizophrenia.

Many people, particularly those concerned with weight loss or heart disease, are fearful of fats. Low-fat diets – which cut down drastically on all types of fat regularly eaten – run a risk of contributing to symptoms of depression and anxiety. Fats matter a lot to emotional and mental health, with low levels in the diet being associated with symptoms that range from anxiety and depression to hyperactivity and schizophrenia.

When you realize that the brain is more than 60 per cent fat it appears to make sense to include some fat in the diet. Fats are essential for the proper structure and functioning of the brain. Many women, for example, have found that by including more of a particular type of essential fat in their diet they have been able to reduce, or remove altogether, the difficult emotional symptoms of premenstrual syndrome. Scientific research is also showing the importance of fat in brain development, its effect on behaviour and for better mental health. So, not all fat is to be avoided, and some fats are even to be encouraged.

When looking at all the different types of food that a person eats, and in particular at the 'fats and oils' group of foods, moderation and balance between the different types of fats is best. (*An explanation of food groups can be found in Chapter 2*). The modern western diet, however, tends to favour certain fats over others with the result that some fats that are essential to emotional and mental health can be overlooked completely.

SATURATED AND UNSATURATED FATS

There are two main types of fat: saturated fats and unsaturated fats. The fats and oils found naturally in foods tend to contain a mixture of saturated and unsaturated fats, with certain foods being higher in one type than another. Saturated fats are higher in animal products such as meat, milk and dairy foods, whereas fish, nuts, seeds and vegetable oils have higher amounts of unsaturated fats. Unsaturated fats are considered to be more healthy than the saturated fats. It is generally agreed that it is best to reduce the amount of saturated fats eaten in favour of having more unsaturated fats.

A third type of fats is the 'trans' or 'hydrogenated' fats. These are modified fats used in margarines, spreads and other processed foods to improve texture and flavour. They are not considered to be supportive of good health in the long term and are best avoided as much as possible.

MONOUNSATURATED AND POLYUNSATURATED FATS

The interest in fats needn't stop here because it is also important to pay attention to the proportions of the different types of unsaturated fats we are eating. Unsaturated fats can be further divided into monounsaturated and polyunsaturated fats. Olive oil which forms the mainstay of the much-praised 'Mediterranean' diet is one example of a food high in monounsaturated fat (also known as oleic acid or 'omega-9' fatty acid). Olive oil is considered to be the best oil for cooking (as well as other uses) because it is the most stable of the unsaturated oils.

Polyunsaturated fats can be divided even further to include two groups of fatty acids known as 'omega-3' (or alpha linolenic acid) and 'omega-6' (or linoleic acid). Omega-3 and omega-6 fatty acids are important essential fatty acids, or 'EFAs', because they cannot be made by the body. They need to be included in a healthy balanced diet. EFAs are vital for good emotional and mental health, being essential for maintaining the structure and proper functioning of brain cell membranes, nerve fibres and neurotransmitters.

ESSENTIAL FATS

Of particular importance for emotional and mental health are the omega-3 essential fats. These are plentiful in oil-rich fish such as mackerel, herring, pilchards, sardines, salmon and fresh tuna. EPA (eicosapentaenoic acid) and DHA (docosahexaenoic acid) are two beneficial omega-3 fats found in fish oils. For those allergic to fish or who are vegetarian or vegan and don't eat fish, the omega-3 essential fatty acids can also be obtained from linseed (flax) oil, pumpkin and hemp seeds and walnuts. The alpha-linolenic (omega-3) fatty acid in these sources can usually be converted by the body into the 'active' fatty acid EPA.

Omega-6 fatty acids are found in vegetable oils such as sunflower and rapeseed oils, which are often used in margarines. They are then converted by the body into a substance called GLA (gamma linolenic acid). Hemp oil contains a small amount of ready-made GLA, as does evening primrose oil.

Essential fats need to be eaten regularly so that the body and brain receive a steady supply of these important nutrients. It is recommended that these good mood fats are eaten at least three times a week or taken daily as a nutritional supplement. The foods that are particularly high in these essential fats are listed in the table below.

♣ Good mood foods include those that contain a relatively higher proportion of unsaturated fats.

- Those high in the omega-3 type of polyunsaturated fat make a particularly good choice.
- For both animal and vegetable sources of omega-3 essential fats, the colder the environment of the food source, the more omega-3 oil it will contain.
- Many people are put off eating fish by the thought of having to deal with fish heads and bones. Although fresh fish is probably best, buying pre-packed fish fillets or tinned fish is both easy and economical. Concerns about the environmental pollution in fish can be counterbalanced by the definite improvements to health that can be experienced within weeks of regularly including a variety of fish in the diet.

Essential Fats in Food

While the precise amounts of nutrients in foods can vary between individual plants or animals, seasons and geographical location, these figures can provide a useful guide to the typical nutrient content of some oil-rich foods.

Vegetarian Food Sources

	Percentage of total fats as polyunsaturated alpha-linolenic acid Omega-3	linoleic acid Omega-6	monounsaturated oleic acid Omega-9	saturated	total fat content
Nuts					
Almonds	–	26%	65%	9%	54%
Brazil nuts	–	24%	48%	24%	67%
Cashew	–	6%	70%	18%	42%
Hazelnut/Filbert	–	16%	54%	5%	62%
Macadamia	–	10%	71%	12%	72%
Peanut	–	29%	47%	18%	48%
Pecan	–	20%	63%	7%	71%
Pistachio	–	19%	65%	9%	54%
Walnut	5%	51%	28%	16%	60%
Seeds					
Flax (linseed)	58%	14%	19%	9%	35%
Hemp	20%	60%	12%	8%	35%

Pumpkin	15%	42%	34%	9%	47%
Sesame	–	45%	42%	13%	49%
Sunflower	–	65%	23%	12%	47%
Other					
Avocado	–	10%	70%	20%	12%
Canola (rapeseed)	7%	30%	54%	7%	30%
Evening primrose	–	81%	11%	8%	17%
Olive	–	8%	76%	16%	20%
Rice bran	1%	35%	48%	17%	10%
Safflower	–	75%	13%	12%	60%
Soybean	7%	50%	26%	15%	18%
Wheatgerm	5%	50%	25%	18%	11%

Fish Sources

Higher levels of omega-3 oils can be found in the following:

- anchovies
- caviar
- eel
- herring
- mackerel
- pilchards
- salmon
- sardines
- trout
- fresh tuna

Good Mood Vitamins and Minerals

Vitamins and minerals are micronutrients that exist in the body in an extremely complex interconnected web of relationships. Without needing to be aware of the particular effects of nutrients or their precise amounts within different foods, by following the general guidelines below you will obtain a balance of many of the vitamins and minerals that are essential for emotional and mental health.

- A diet that contains plenty of fresh fruit and vegetables will provide many nutrients essential for good mental health. It is recommended that we eat at least five portions of fruit and vegetables every day – and that doesn't include potatoes! Although fresh is usually considered best, frozen fruit and vegetables can often provide an acceptable alternative, often containing levels of nutrients comparable to fresh produce.

- Imbalances in vitamins and minerals can result from a build-up of environmental toxins. Choosing organically-grown foods reduces this risk.
- Wholefoods that are unrefined, with the minimum processing possible, can contain higher levels of vital vitamins, minerals and essential fatty acids.
- Eating a diet that is as varied as possible, where the variety is spread out over several days (rather than crammed into one day), ensures a better balance of micronutrients.

Research is revealing specific micronutrients that appear to be important for emotional and mental health.

Research is revealing specific micronutrients that appear to be important for emotional and mental health. The significance of certain nutrients and their relationship with how we feel is an area of knowledge that is continually evolving. The list of vitamins and minerals below gives some of the nutrients which have been found as particularly important for emotional and mental health. They are listed together with examples of how they may be needed, to give a flavour of why they are considered to be so important. Some good food sources of these nutrients are also provided.

ANTIOXIDANTS

These are nutrients that can counter the negative effects of harmful 'free radicals'. Free radicals are electron-hungry molecules which are formed in the body as a consequence of being exposed to different stressors such as alcohol, fried food, pollution, stress and smoking. Free radicals create oxidative stress and cause damage to cells in the body and brain. Vitamins A, C and E, beta-carotene and the mineral selenium, plus many other plant substances including bioflavonoids, are the best-known substances which have been found to have a beneficial antioxidant effect. Vitamin C helps with the conversion of tryptophan to serotonin.

Some good food sources of antioxidant vitamins include:

- dried apricots
- almonds
- avocado
- beans
- berries
- blackcurrants
- broccoli
- Brussels sprouts
- liver (and fish liver oil)
- mango
- melon
- oranges
- organ meats
- papaya
- pumpkin
- red and green sweet peppers

- cabbage
- carrots
- cashew nuts
- cauliflower
- citrus fruit
- eggs
- hazelnuts
- kiwi fruit

- seeds
- spinach
- sweet potato
- tangerines
- tomatoes
- vegetable oils
- walnuts
- watercress

Selenium is found in:

- brazil nuts
- cabbage
- chicken
- courgettes (zucchini)
- herring

- seafood
- sesame seeds
- sunflower seeds
- tuna
- whole grains

B-VITAMINS AND FOLIC ACID (FOLATE)

These nutrients are often grouped together because of the similarities in the way they work. There are certain B-vitamins that appear particularly important for their ability to improve energy, mood and mental functioning. For example, vitamin B_3 (niacin) has been found to be deficient in some cases of schizophrenia; B_5 (pantothenic acid) is required for stress hormones and the neurotransmitter associated with memory, acetylcholine. Vitamin B_6 (pyridoxine) is an important co-factor (helper nutrient) in the metabolism of essential fatty acids and the production of the neurotransmitter serotonin. It has also received particular attention for its benefit in the treatment of premenstrual syndrome. Vitamin B_{12} is vital for a healthy nervous system as is folic acid (folate), and low levels of both these nutrients have been associated with dementia and depression in the elderly.

Some good food sources of B-vitamins include:

- avocados
- bananas
- beans
- carrots
- eggs
- fish (e.g. salmon, tuna)
- lentils

- meat
- milk
- molasses
- nuts (e.g. almonds, cashew nuts)
- seeds (e.g. sunflower seeds)
- whole grains (e.g. brown rice)
- yeast

MAGNESIUM

Magnesium is another co-factor in the metabolism (processing) of essential fatty acids. Low levels of magnesium can be associated with nervous tension, anxiety, irritability, hyperactivity and insomnia.

Some good food sources of magnesium include:

- leafy green vegetables
- nuts (such as brazil nuts, almonds,
- hazelnuts and peanuts)
- whole grains (particularly millet and oats)

MANGANESE

Manganese is another co-factor for fatty acid synthesis. Insufficient manganese may be a contributory factor in schizophrenia, other psychotic disorders and also epilepsy.

Some good food sources of manganese include:

- beetroot
- blackberries
- celery
- grapes
- lettuce
- lima (butter) beans
- oats
- pineapple
- raspberries
- strawberries
- watercress

POTASSIUM

Potassium is important for maintaining a correct acid–alkali balance in the body and for maintaining a healthy nervous system.

Some good food sources of potassium include:

- apricots
- almonds
- avocado
- bananas
- beans
- cabbage
- cashew nuts
- cauliflower
- celery
- courgettes (zucchini)
- melon
- molasses
- mushrooms
- parsley
- pumpkin
- radishes
- sunflower seeds
- watercress

ZINC

A common mineral to be deficient in, zinc appears to be a critical nutrient for good mental and emotional health and the need for zinc increases during times of stress. Zinc is an important co-factor for the metabolism of essential fatty acids and the production of the neurotransmitter serotonin. It is also important for maintaining the integrity of the blood–brain barrier. Low levels of zinc are also associated with a wide range of symptoms including anxiety and depression, and mental illnesses from anorexia and bulimia to schizophrenia. Some forms of schizophrenia can be due to pyroluria which is an unusually high requirement for zinc and vitamin B_6.

Some good food sources of zinc include:

- brazil nuts
- herring
- lamb
- meats
- oysters
- pumpkin seeds
- sesame seeds
- sunflower seeds
- walnuts
- whole grains

AMINO ACIDS

As well as occurring naturally in protein foods, amino acids can be taken in supplement form to boost abnormally low levels. Amino acids can themselves function as brain chemicals and are also precursors (parent nutrients) for some neurotransmitters. Some amino acids essential for mental and emotional functioning include:

- Arginine (which may increase brain blood flow and neurotransmitter nitric oxide levels and reduce oxidative stress).
- Glutamine (which is the precursor for GABA, gamma-aminobutyric acid, an important inhibitory neurotransmitter).
- Glycine (which can decrease cravings for sugar and alcohol and reduce feelings of aggression and anxiety).
- Histidine (which is needed for histamine formation required for sexual arousal).
- Methionine (which helps detoxify heavy metals from the brain and also excess histamine). Methionine is metabolized to s-adenosyl-methionine (SAMe).
- Phenylalanine (which stimulates production of cholecystokinin (CCK) for appetite control and is also needed for the production of tyrosine).
- Pyroglutamate (which is needed for learning and memory).
- Tryptophan (which is converted into serotonin, the calming neurotransmitter needed for appetite control, good moods and sleep).

♣ Tyrosine (which forms the 'arousing' neurotransmitters dopamine, noradrenalin (norepinephrine) and adrenalin (epinephrine)).

There are other amino acids that influence the functioning of the brain and, as with all nutrients, it is necessary to get the correct balance between all amino acids.

Case Study: Breakdown

Suzannah was aged 45, divorced and attempting to regain her health and resume her career in publishing. She had been on chlorpromazine, an anti-psychotic drug, for 20 years and had had several psychotic breakdowns. The symptoms of mental illness had begun following the breakdown of her very unhappy marriage. Suzannah had suffered two severe post-natal depressions after her children were born, and during the second episode was hospitalized and separated from her children. She was put on chlorpromazine and received ECT (electro-convulsive therapy) treatments. Then she started to experience paranoia.

When Suzannah consulted a nutritional therapist she was wanting to come off her medication as she believed it was contributing to her insomnia. She was also beginning to suffer from symptoms of trembling known as tardive dyskinesia, a recognized side-effect of the long-term use of chlorpromazine. Suzannah was 'very frightened', however, that she would become psychotic on giving up the medication, as she had done in the past.

Suzannah was recommended to remain on her medication for the time being and try a gluten-free diet (that is no wheat, oats, rye, barley or spelt). It was suggested she gave up drinking her six to eight daily cups of tea and coffee. She was advised to cut down on refined foods and sugar in order to improve her blood sugar metabolism and to cut down on yeast-containing foods to relieve a likely yeast sensitivity. An organic whole food diet was recommended, high in raw vegetables and fruit, plus plenty of water. Her nutritional therapist also prescribed a personal nutritional supplement programme that consisted of a good quality multivitamin and mineral supplement and essential fats such as evening primrose oil, plus additional vitamins and minerals which were indicated as being necessary for her to take.

Within a year of making these changes to her diet and starting the supplement programme she was able to get, and hold down, a new and very demanding job. She now felt so well, slept through the night and had so much energy that she felt confident enough to give up her medication. Four years later, Suzannah has gone from strength to strength in her health and her career. She describes herself as 'emotionally stable' and is 'embracing life to the full'. Suzannah has shown no signs of her former anxiety, depression, paranoia or psychosis. The 'diet' became integrated into her daily routine as a new way of life and she is still following her supplement programme. Suzannah says that she has 'regained the health and stamina she had lost' and she has recently remarried.

Nutrients in the Mind Meal

The ingredients of the Mind Meal contain many important nutrients, some of which are shown below. Those listed are particularly important for emotional and mental health and can be found at relatively higher levels in the foods indicated.

	Omega-3 fats	Antioxidants	B-vits	Magnesium	Manganese	Potassium	Zinc	Tryptophan
wheat-free pasta			✓	✓				
pesto sauce			✓	✓		✓		
oil-rich fish	✓		✓					✓
mixed green salad		✓	✓	✓		✓		
avocado		✓	✓		✓			✓
sunflower seeds			✓			✓	✓	✓
pumpkin seeds	✓		✓			✓	✓	✓
bananas			✓			✓		
dried apricots		✓	✓	✓		✓		✓
oatcakes			✓	✓	✓	✓		
walnuts	✓		✓	✓		✓		✓

Fats, Carbohydrates and Protein

These three major components of food are all needed for good emotional and mental health.

FATS

The brain is over 60 per cent fat. Avoiding all types of fat – in a low-fat diet for example – can lead to anxiety and depression and other mental health problems. Polyunsaturated 'omega-3' fats are particularly important. These are found in oil-rich fish, nuts and seeds and need to be eaten several times every week.

PROTEIN

This is made up of fragments known as amino acids. Some amino acids can have a direct effect on levels of certain brain chemicals. For example, eating foods naturally high in tryptophan can improve mood as the tryptophan is converted by the body to serotonin, an important brain chemical that regulates impulse control and appetite, elevates mood, self-esteem, feelings of optimism and induces calm feelings and sleep.

CARBOHYDRATE

The absorption of tryptophan into the brain is greatly enhanced by eating carbohydrate-containing foods, and carbohydrate cravings can be explained as a subconscious drive to increase serotonin levels *(see also Chapters 2, 3 and 8).*

FOOD COMBINING

Although those with a sluggish digestive system may benefit from eating protein- and carbohydrate-containing foods at different meals (as is the practice in food-combining diets, for example), there are potential problems associated with this way of eating. If overall protein intake is reduced then the amount of tryptophan eaten will also be less. Also, cutting down on the frequency of eating starchy foods reduces the frequency of the tryptophan-absorbing effect of carbohydrates. Low levels of tryptophan may result in lower serotonin levels and symptoms such as food cravings or depression. Protein and carbohydrate eaten together results in a slower release of energy from food. A slow energy release avoids the highs and subsequent dips in mood and energy that can follow a carbohydrate-concentrated meal.

The Value of Water

If you change only one thing in your diet you could do a lot worse than simply increasing the amount of plain water you drink

If you change only one thing in your diet you could do a lot worse than simply increasing the amount of plain water you drink, for water can have a profound effect on the way we feel. Symptoms of 'fuzzy thinking' and poor concentration, for example, can simply be a matter of dehydration which is soon improved by having a glass of water. Water is also the solvent for many of the toxins that are flushed out of the body in the urine via the kidneys. When reducing the amount of caffeine you consume, withdrawal symptoms such as headaches can be helped by increasing the amount of water that is drunk throughout the day.

The body is approximately three-quarters water. About two litres, or approximately eight tumblers, of water are needed every day to replace fluids excreted in waste products, sweat and even in the air we exhale. More than this amount is needed in warmer weather and when undertaking physical exercise. If your urine is darker in colour with a strong smell, then dehydration is the likely cause. Counting the water which is used in cups of tea or coffee towards your total water intake doesn't work, as the caffeine contained in these drinks has a diuretic effect, causing you to get rid of yet more water. Diluted fruit juices, for example, are better than no water-containing liquids at all, but drinking plain water is the most effective solution for dehydration.

Although many people do not actually feel thirsty, most of us appear to be suffering from chronic dehydration to some degree and feel better if we drink more water. Beginning a regime of drinking more water may take a certain amount of discipline – even willpower. Nevertheless, the benefits to the way you think and feel can appear within a week or two of making a concerted effort to drink more water. Eventually, your thirst sensation will be reawakened and plain water will become the thirst-quenching drink you enjoy.

Water-drinking Tips

♣ Warm water can be more pleasant to drink than cold – especially in winter – and is less of a 'shock' to the stomach. On occasions, try drinking just warm water from the kettle instead of your usual cup of tea or coffee.

♣ Plain water can be livened up with a slice of lemon – but not if you have a sensitivity to citrus fruit!

♣ Starting the day with a drink of water supports your body in flushing out the toxins that have been building up during your overnight fast. This healthy habit can also be used to encourage the regular bowel motions that help with healthy brain functioning.

♣ If you dislike the taste of tap water, try bottled water or water that has been filtered through a filter jug or undersink unit. This can also benefit those who are sensitive to the chemicals in tap water that are not found in the bottled or filtered alternatives.

♣ Aim to have the majority of your water intake away from meals. Large quantities of water drunk at mealtimes can dilute the digestive juices, making them less effective.

♣ Plan water-stops throughout the day to ensure you reach your daily target of two litres or eight tumblers. You could draw a chart to record each time you drink some water. Or you could fill a large bottle with water each morning and then watch how the level goes down as you drink its contents during the day.

Water-bathing Tip

Nutrients can be absorbed through the skin and bathing in sulphur-rich spas has long known to be beneficial for health. Adding a capful of Epsom salts (magnesium sulphate) to the bath water is one way of increasing sulphate levels in the body. Sulphation affects many processes including the metabolism of certain neurotransmitters and the integrity of the gut lining and is thought to be a key consideration in the cause of autism.

Good Mood Herbs

Many common herbs which are used in cooking for their flavour and aroma can also be included in recipes for their effects on the mind. Other herbs, such as chamomile (which has a calming effect and can help with insomnia), are usually taken in the form of a tea. Herbal teas are available in many food stores and can be purchased as loose tea or tea bags. They can be used as alternatives to tea and coffee and do not contain caffeine.

Also available are concentrated herbal preparations which are used specifically for their therapeutic benefits for emotional and mental health. For example, herbs such as St John's Wort (*Hypericum perforatum*) or Kava Kava (*Piper methysticum*) can be used to help symptoms of depression and anxiety respectively. However, if you are already taking any medication, it is essential that you first consult your doctor for guidance prior to trying these herbal remedies. It is very unwise to suddenly stop taking any medication, and if you continue with some drugs whilst also taking herbal remedies, the combination can create unpleasant side-effects. It is also recommended that you consult a medical herbalist about using these herbs, which don't necessarily suit everyone.

Knowledge of the benefits of herbs for the mind comes from their use down the ages in traditional folk medicine as well as in the modern-day practices of herbalism and aromatherapy (which uses essential oils extracted from herbs). The herbs listed here are some that can be used in cooking or to make a tea for drinking.

BASIL

Can have a clarifying effect on the mind, sharpen the senses and improve concentration. Used in cooking, it works particularly well with tomatoes or to make pesto sauce.

CHAMOMILE

A soothing herb that helps to ease anxiety and tension and promotes relaxation. Can be of benefit for insomnia. The dried herb is usually used loose or in bags to make a tea.

CINNAMON

A spice that can help counteract exhaustion, fatigue and weakness. May help with depression. It also appears to have an insulin-enhancing effect and may help regulate blood sugar levels. Used in baking and with cooked fruit such as apples and pears.

CORIANDER/CILANTRO

Reputed to have a refreshing, stimulating and uplifting effect on the mind and may help with lethargy and tension. The leaves or seeds may be used in a variety of cooked dishes.

GINGER

A warming and stimulating herb that can lift the spirits and ease depression. Can be used in cooking in many ways and, by adding boiling water, taken as a warming drink.

GINGKO

Can be taken as a tea for age-related memory decline and also to counter the reduction in libido that is a side-effect of certain antidepressant medication.

KAVA KAVA

A member of the pepper family, particularly effective for symptoms of anxiety. Also helpful for insomnia, stress and depression. Can be taken as a tea.

LEMON BALM

A herb used as a tea. Good for anxiety and irritability. Can help with insomnia.

MARJORAM

Helpful for calming the nervous system and reducing anxiety and feelings of stress. Can be used in cooking and the fresh herb may be added to salads.

PEPPERMINT

A cooling herb that can reduce angry feelings and nervousness. It can also help with mental fatigue. Often used with vegetables and salads or drunk in the form of a refreshing tea which can be enjoyed hot or chilled.

ROSEMARY

A stimulating herb, reputedly good for improving the memory. Used in cooking and can be sprinkled over roasted vegetables and meats.

ST JOHN'S WORT

Excellent reputation for the treatment of depression. Can also help with anxiety, insomnia and SAD (seasonal affective disorder). Can be taken as a tea.

VALERIAN

May be taken as a tea to help with sleep problems. Can also benefit anxiety, depression and stress.

Taking Nutritional Supplements

Many psychological symptoms can be linked to nutritional deficiencies which, when treated with nutritional supplements, can improve dramatically.

Many psychological symptoms can be linked to nutritional deficiencies which, when treated with nutritional supplements, can improve dramatically. Of course, taking supplements is no substitute for eating a varied and balanced diet containing plenty of fresh fruit and vegetables. Other lifestyle considerations (such as exercise and relaxation) are also essential ingredients in the recipe for good mental health. However, regular supplementation can provide protection against deficiencies arising from erratic eating, illnesses which require additional nutritional support and the effects of environmental pollution. Supplements can also help to redress the imbalances caused by foods that contain artificial chemicals or which are of a poor nutritional quality.

Compared to the effort required in changing your diet, taking nutritional supplements has the advantage of involving the least disruption to daily life. Taking supplements and changing your diet at the same time is likely to achieve the greatest gains in the least amount of time. A disadvantage of doing several things at once to improve your health is that you then cannot be certain which change is having which benefit.

Tips for Taking Nutritional Supplements

1 The best source of vitamins and minerals is a varied diet containing plenty of fresh fruit and vegetables, whole grains, meat and fish. However, your need for certain nutrients may be greater, which means you will need to make up a deficit through taking nutritional supplements.

2 Nutritional supplements can be purchased from a health-food store, pharmacist or general food stores. If you have a sympathetic doctor, it may be possible for you to get some supplements on prescription.

3 If you can afford to take only one supplement, take a quality multivitamin and mineral supplement. This may be all you need to redress nutritional imbalances, correct faulty biochemistry and support the body's detoxification processes. A 'multi' also provides a firm foundation before 'topping up' with other nutrients, if and when these are needed. Different 'multis' tend to vary in their combination of nutrients. It may be worth periodically changing your supplement to benefit from the different emphasis of each formula.

4 Particularly beneficial good mood nutrients include the B-group vitamins and the minerals magnesium and zinc. These will be included in a 'multi' but you may need to top up with more of these nutrients *(but see 7 below)*.

5 Buy the best supplements you can afford. If shopping around for a bargain and comparing products, make sure you read the labels to compare the actual amounts of each nutrient. Bioavailability – how easily your body can absorb and use the nutrients – is an important consideration and generally worth paying for.

6 Essential fats, particularly those found in oil-rich fish and linseed/flax oil, are available in supplement form and are important to include, especially if these foods are not eaten several times each week.

7 It is important to get the correct balance between different vitamins and minerals and to avoid taking any one nutrient in excess. A good quality multivitamin and mineral supplement should contain nutrients in a carefully balanced formulation. Overdosing on supplements is possible if you start to 'pick and mix' individual supplements without reading further or asking professional advice. Assessing your need for supplements is best done by a nutritional therapist who can then recommend a supplement programme designed to meet your specific needs.

8 There are so many supplements now available, with new products coming on to the market virtually every week, that it's easy to become caught up in the belief that 'more' means 'better'. It is also easy to end up spending more than you may be able to afford so you could decide to have a limited budget that controls your spending on supplements. To help keep within spending limits you could designate an amount for 'essential' supplementation, such as a good quality 'multi', and use the remainder of your allowance for experimenting with new products, as and when they seem appropriate.

Food–Mood–Medicine Interactions

Certain medications, nutritional supplements, herbal supplements and foods can all interact and occasionally create potentially harmful side-effects or reduce the effectiveness of medication. If you are taking any medication it is wise to check with your doctor or nutritional therapist about the possibility of interactions before starting a nutritional supplement programme or taking any herbal remedies. Interactions between food and medications are also possible, and as far as mood medication is concerned, it is important to be aware of the risk of reactions occurring between the MAOI (monoamine oxidase inhibitor) type of antidepressant and a naturally-occurring substance in some foods called tyramine.

The interaction between MAOIs and tyramine can cause dangerous rises in blood pressure which may be signalled by a throbbing headache. Foods containing particularly high levels of tyramine and which must be avoided when on this type of medication include:

- broad beans
- yeast extract
- meat extract
- fermented soya bean extract
- salted, smoked or pickled fish (especially pickled herring)
- most cheeses.

As the action of bacteria on protein produces tyramine, MAOI users are advised to avoid stale food or food which may be 'going off'. This is particularly relevant for protein-rich foods such as meat, fish or chicken; game meats should be avoided completely. A full list of tyramine-containing foods can be obtained from your doctor or nutritional therapist.

Good Mood Food Checklist

- Low in (or free from) added sugar
- Low in (or free from) caffeine
- Low in (or free from) artificial additives
- Hypoallergenic (i.e. low or free from foods, such as wheat and milk, that you have confirmed provoke sensitivity reactions)
- Low to medium Glycaemic Index
- Contains nutrients for mental health

Low Sugar

Sugar sensitivity is often associated with symptoms of aggression, anxiety, confusion, poor concentration, depression, fatigue and irritability. These symptoms are often reduced when foods containing added sugars are avoided. *For more information see Chapter 8.*

Low Caffeine

Cutting down on stimulants such as caffeine – found in coffee, tea, chocolate and cola – reduces the highs and the subsequent lows associated with the use of these foods and drinks, making for a smoother emotional ride through the day. *For more information see Chapter 7.*

Low Additives

Additives, particularly artificial colourings, can be found associated with behaviour-disturbing symptoms including attention deficit disorder and hyperactivity. *A list of additives to avoid is provided in Chapter 6.*

Hypoallergenic

Many frequently-eaten foods can be linked to moods, and reducing the amount consumed can result in dramatic improvements in health. Common offenders are wheat (found in most breads, pastas and pizzas) and milk (plus butter, cheese and yoghurt). *For more information on this aspect of mood food, see Chapters 4 to 6.*

Low Glycaemic Index

Eating foods and meals with a low to medium GI, which release their energy slowly, also helps to avoid the roller-coaster ride of energy and moods associated with large fluctuations in blood glucose levels. *For more information see Chapter 8.*

'Good Mood' Nutrients

Low levels of certain nutrients have been associated with various symptoms of mental illness including anxiety, depression and even schizophrenia. Essential nutrients to look for in foods are the omega-3 fatty acids found in oil-rich fish and also in some nuts and seeds. Also particularly important for mental health are the B-vitamins and the minerals zinc, magnesium and selenium. Eating foods naturally high in tryptophan, an amino acid found in protein, can also improve mood, and its absorption is assisted by eating carbohydrate foods.

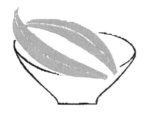

10

Shopping and C-king

Despite the abundance of cooking programmes on television and the countless magazine pages devoted to recipes and eating, to 'cook' remains, for many, an unappealing four-letter word. Cooking in any form is the culmination of planning, shopping, and food preparation. It is almost certain that what, when and how we choose to cook expresses the many feelings we have about food and eating.

Successful Change

Changing what you eat to improve the way you feel can lead you to a different way of thinking about food. To begin, you become *aware* of food's power to affect your emotions and the functioning of your mind. Then, by experimenting with the ideas in this handbook, you discover the possible benefits to your health. Finally, you integrate into your daily routine the changes that work for you, placing a new emphasis on the importance of food.

The *availability* of the food you need is crucial to the success of any changes you hope to make.

On a more practical level, you will need to decide which foods are *acceptable* to you and which are compatible with your way of life. The *availability* of the food you need is crucial to the success of any changes you hope to make. So, finding out where to obtain what you need and the accessibility of supplies will be essential groundwork. The 'Where to Go?' section later in this chapter contains some suggestions for finding what you need.

Affordability is something that should be considered carefully. Some foods on your shopping list may now be more expensive, but you will be able to cut back in other areas. Choosing more fresh fruit and vegetables, for example, to eat as quick and tasty snacks, may appear to be an extra expense but savings are then likely – perhaps as you reduce the amount of biscuits you buy. When calculating the cost of making changes, you'll need to set them against the benefit of improvements to your emotional and mental health. It can be difficult to place a price on better health, but the overall feeling should be that any costs, together with your efforts, have all been worthwhile.

Having become more aware of the effect of food on mood, and considered the acceptability, availability and affordability of alternative foods, all that remains is to ensure that what you eat *appeals* to your taste buds. If food doesn't taste good, and you don't enjoy eating it, this will surely affect your mood – but for the worse! To help you, this chapter offers a week's worth of good mood meal suggestions together with signposts directing you to even more good mood food ideas.

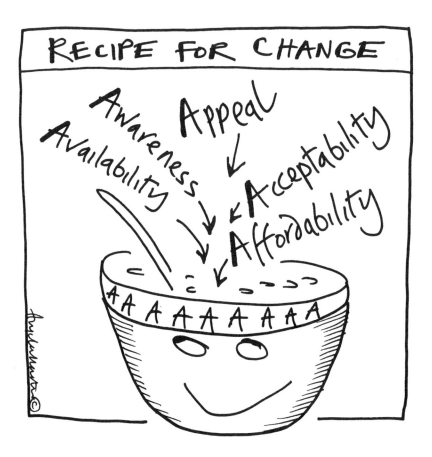

Fig 26 – Recipe for change

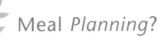

Meal *Planning*?

Food, for many people, comes near the bottom of the list of 'things to do', and at the end of the day, preparing dinner is often a chore to be endured whilst feeling tired and irritable.

Whatever your level of income, life in the 21st century seems to be faster and busier with too many competing demands. Food, for many people, comes near the bottom of the list of 'things to do', and at the end of the day, preparing dinner is often a chore to be endured whilst feeling tired and irritable. In the stress-filled world we inhabit, food seems to be used ever more as the carrot and the stick – a means of reward and control. It seems that life is good only if there is something satisfying to eat after a hard day's work. If we can bribe others with culinary treats, or reward ourselves with food, then so much the better.

Meals, it seems, are often thought of on the basis of the type of foods they contain. When planning what to have for breakfast, most people will be thinking along the lines of 'cereal, toast and a drink' rather than a food's protein, carbohydrate, fat and fibre content. There probably won't have been a second thought given to the meal's ingredients, such as whether it contains wheat, cow's milk or caffeine. Lunch is often chosen on the basis of its convenience, portability and speed. (This is where sandwiches, soup, crisps and chocolate often show up as favourites.) Then, when it comes to dinner, it is usually a question of something that, once again, is quick and easy. Appeal to the taste buds is, of course, essential – in order to 'make up for' the stresses and strains of the day.

So, with all this in mind, this chapter aims to approach meal planning in a way that makes sense for how most people think about food. A useful method is to use the food plate idea (*introduced in Chapter 2*) which tends to reflect the way most people shop for food and prepare meals. If you are wanting to try a rotation diet then the food plate can also form a guide to help you plan a balanced rotation of foods. (*The advantages of rotating foods are described in Chapter 6, together with a step-by-step approach for devising a rotation diet.*)

Chapter 9 contains details of the Mind Meal, a three-course example of how to use some good mood foods. Here you will also find a good mood food checklist to guide you in your food choices. You may also like to try out the quick-and-easy good mood recipes which are scattered throughout this handbook. The Resources section at the end provides details of some excellent cookbooks which have been written with special diets in mind.

Good Mood Food Plate

The food plate approach to meal planning recommends we eat food from each of the segments of the plate every day. The size of the segments shows roughly how much of that food we need to eat, compared to the other foods that make up the rest of the plate. The food plate given here has taken into account the possibility of food sensitivities and the need to find alternative and substitute foods to eat instead. You can see that there is plenty to choose from, and as general awareness of alternative foods grows, more choices will become available.

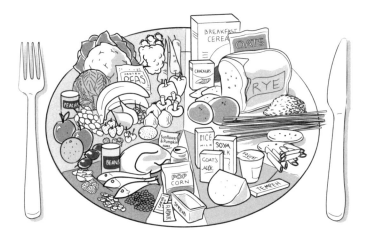

Fig 27 – Good Mood Food Plate

FRUIT AND VEGETABLES

This section makes up about one-third of the foods you eat. The minimum recommended amount of fruit and vegetables is five portions every day. The information on food families in Chapter 6 can guide you on any possible cross-reactions with close relatives of a particular fruit or vegetable. The food families list can also be used as a checklist of foods to try, in order to increase the variety of what you eat.

STARCHY STAPLES

This section also makes up about one-third of the foods you eat. For someone who wants to avoid wheat – one of the most common foods for people to be sensitive to – there are many wheat-free alternatives available. So, this section includes wheat-free breakfast cereals such as cornflakes, puffed rice and porridge oats. Then there are wheat-free breads such as rye bread, pumpernickel and corn bread; grains such as rice, millet, quinoa, buckwheat, polenta (made from corn/maize); wheat-free pastas such as buckwheat pasta or corn spaghetti and crackers such as oatcakes, rice cakes and rye crackers. This section of the 'plate' includes starchy root vegetables such as white potatoes, sweet potato and yam.

The remaining three sections together make up the final third of the plate.

MEAT, FISH AND ALTERNATIVES

This section can also include vegetarian substitutes for meat made from soya or myco-protein. The healthier way to eat soya is as part of a rotation diet and in the form of fermented soya products such as tempeh and miso. Other protein foods include members of the legume family such as beans, peas and lentils. Nuts and seeds could also be included here for their protein content.

MILK AND DAIRY FOODS

If you want to avoid cow's milk (and products made from this milk) there are a number of alternatives available. Goat's and sheep's milk are two alternatives that may suit some people. Otherwise, choose from soya milk, rice milk, oat milk, pea milk, almond milk and other 'milks' made from nuts and seeds. Apart from goat's milk, these cow's milk substitutes are not suitable for children under the age of two years. If you would like to change your child's diet you are advised to consult a nutritional therapist first.

If you can get calcium-enriched milk alternatives, so much the better. It is wise to make sure you include plenty of calcium- and magnesium-rich foods in your diet (such as tinned fish with edible bones, leafy green vegetables, nuts such as brazil nuts, almonds, hazelnuts and peanuts and whole grains, particularly millet and oats). You could also take a nutritional supplement that contains these minerals.

The main substitute for cow's milk yoghurts (apart from those made from goat's or sheep's milk) is soya yoghurt. Other alternatives such as yoghurt made from oat milk is not so easily available and you may need to think of other desserts to substitute instead. These could include fresh fruit or perhaps the 'rice flake delight' (*see recipe, page 206*).

FAT AND SUGAR

These foods make up the smallest segment on the plate. The importance of including healthy polyunsaturated fats rather than saturated, trans or hydrogenated fats is discussed in Chapter 9. Information on the need to choose slow-releasing sugar-containing foods can be found in Chapter 8. This segment of the 'food plate' can include milk-free and/or soya-free margarines instead of butter and spreads containing hydrogenated/trans fats. Olive oil drizzled over bread can be used as an alternative to butter or margarine. Tasty alternative snacks and treats include carob bars, corn chips/crisps, popcorn, bags of nuts and dried fruit mixes, flapjacks, oatcakes with sugar- and sweetener-free jam/fruit spread/honey, and cakes and biscuits made with wheat-free flour. For fun sweet-tasting drinks, choose from the variety of fruit juices diluted with carbonated water that are now available as canned drinks. Of course, these can be made at home very easily and more economically by combining fruit juice and carbonated spring water.

Milk and Alternatives: a Comparison of Nutrients (per 100ml)

The information in this table has been compiled from a variety of sources including food manufacturers and suppliers, and is intended only as a guide to nutrient levels. Some alternative milks are not appropriate for young children and professional advice should be obtained regarding suitable milk substitutes.

Nutrient	Human	Cow	Goat	Ewe	Buffalo	Soya	Rice	Oat	Almond	Pea
energy (kcal)	69.00	66.00	61.00	95.00	111.00	32.00	51.00	42.00	51.80	51.00
protein (g)	2.00	3.20	3.10	5.40	4.5	2.4	0.42	1.0	1.0	3.2
fat (g)	4.10	3.90	3.50	6.00	8.0	1.3	0.84	1.5	2.5	3.4
carbohydrate (g)	7.20	4.80	4.40	5.10	4.9	2.8	10.42	6.5	6.32	1.8
calcium (mg)	34.00	120.00	100.00	170.00	195.00	128.00*	125.00*	–	–	42.00

* nutrient content of calcium-enriched version

– figures not available

Where to Go?

Availability of food is fundamental to making changes to what you eat. The following is an alphabetical list of suggestions for where to find what you need.

Buyers' Groups

If availability and affordability in your area are a problem then one solution is to form a buyers' group. All this takes is a group of people who want to eat food that is not easily available in their local stores. The group gets together to buy in bulk and to have access to a wholesaler. Alternative food suppliers are often quite happy to make a delivery to a group of individuals living in an area where there are no other retail outlets for their products.

Delicatessens

These specialist stores are a source of foods sometimes not available in general food stores. Unusual milks and cheeses and wheat-free pastas, for example, can often be found here, although prices are usually somewhat higher.

Doctors and Pharmacists

Some 'special diet' foods, such as gluten-free bread, are available on prescription through doctors. There are, however, strict guidelines as to which health conditions justify providing food on prescription, and obtaining special food in this way is restricted. Pharmacists may sell 'special diet' foods or can place an order on your behalf, without the need for a prescription. Be warned, however, that these 'special diet' foods tend to be very expensive.

General Food Stores

As awareness of the need for alternative foods that cater for special diets grows, general food stores are increasing their range of produce. Larger stores can usually provide customers with information on which items are suitable for their particular dietary needs.

Basmati Rice with Flaked Fish and Green Peas

Type: Lunch/Dinner
Equipment: Medium pan, hob
Preparation time: 5 mins
Cooking time: 20 mins

Basmati rice contains a higher proportion of the slowly-digested amylose starch. This means it has a particularly low Glycaemic Index and makes a good choice for a carbohydrate that won't create a blood sugar high to be followed by a rebound low. Oil-rich fish from a tin are an excellent, easy and economical source of the beneficial omega-3 essential fats needed to 'oil the brain'. A balance in colour is provided with something green so peas seem the ideal choice for this recipe. Frozen peas (also having a low GI) are very convenient. The freezing of vegetables retains high vitamin levels which can so easily be reduced in the not-so-fresh alternatives.

Ingredients (per person)

75g/3oz/1/2 cup basmati rice
1 small tin oil-rich fish in brine/spring water or olive oil e.g. mackerel, salmon, sardines, pilchards or fresh tuna
75g/3oz/1/2 cup frozen peas

Method

1   Rinse and cook the rice according to the instructions on the packet.
2   Meanwhile, drain the liquid from the tinned fish, tip into a bowl and flake with a fork. Large bones can be removed but smaller bones are soft, edible and a good source of calcium.
3   Cook the frozen peas in a pan of boiling water for 5 mins, then drain.
4   When rice is ready, drain and tip into a bowl. Add the fish and peas and fold gently together.
5   Serve. If liked, plain live soya yoghurt can be used as a dressing.

Ready?	The only ingredient to watch in this recipe is the rice which you can sample to see if it is ready or not.
Underdone	Still crunchy.
Just right	Just soft enough to eat and grains not sticking together.
Overdone	Rice that is overdone tends to stick together (*see below*).
Trouble-shooting tip	Overdone rice provides the ideal base for making rice 'balls' or 'patties'. In this recipe the ingredients can be combined in a bowl and then squeezed into small balls which can then be flattened slightly and grilled. Alternatively, the mixture could be pressed into an oven-proof dish and browned in the oven to create a rice-fish 'bake'.

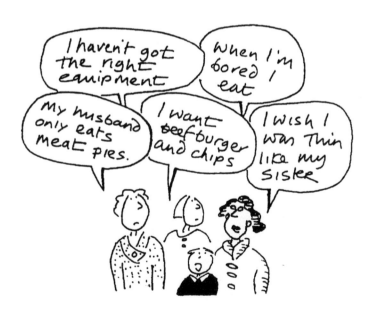

'Green Box' Schemes

Green box schemes cater for those who wish to buy seasonal organic fruit and vegetables from a local supplier. A good value selection of fresh produce can be delivered weekly although there isn't always a choice of what you get in your 'box'. Some schemes also offer meat, fish, eggs and dried goods.

Health-food Stores

Specialist health-food stores are the obvious place to shop for alternative foods and ingredients. They invariably offer nutritional supplements as well and may also sell special diet cookbooks.

Internet Shopping

Home shopping is available on the internet where general and specialist food suppliers can be found. An internet home delivery service is also offered by many larger food stores.

Mail Order

Some food producers such as farmers or bakers sell their wares direct to the public via a mail order service.

Markets and Farmers' Markets

Markets are a source of fresh, often locally grown, produce at reasonable prices. They often have a lively atmosphere and provide an opportunity to enjoy shopping in a different environment.

Some Suggested Alternatives

Listed below are some more unusual alternatives you could substitute for your problem foods. There are also some ideas for how these alternatives can be used.

Alternative food	Buy as	Use as/for
Amaranth	grain	rice
	puffs	breakfast cereal/topping
Buckwheat	flakes	porridge/muesli
	flour	pancakes, sauces
	groats/kasha	rice
	noodles	noodles
	pasta	pasta
	puffed	breakfast cereal
Corn (maize)	bread	toast
	chips/crisps	snack
	flakes	breakfast cereal
	flour	baking/sauces
	kernels	making popcorn
	meal	baking/sauces
	on-the-cob	snack/starter
	pasta	pasta
	polenta	mashed potato cakes
	puffs	breakfast cereal
	spaghetti	spaghetti
	sweetcorn	a vegetable
	tacos	container for 'mince' or vegetables
	tortillas	container for 'mince' or vegetables
Millet	flakes	porridge/muesli
	flour	baking/pancakes
	grain	rice
	puffs	breakfast cereal/topping
Oats	cakes	biscuits/crackers
	grain	stews/casseroles
	rolled	porridge

Quinoa	flakes	porridge/muesli
	grain	rice
Rice	cakes	crackers
	crackers	crackers
	flakes	cereal/porridge/pudding
	grain	rice
	flour	baking/sauces/batters
	puffs	rice 'krispies' breakfast cereal/cakes
Rye	bread	bread
	flour	baking/batters
	grain	stews/casseroles/sprouting
	pumpernickel	toast
Soya	beans	a bean
	cheese	cheese
	cream	cream
	flour	baking/pancakes
	margarine	margarine/butter
	milk	milk
	miso (with barley/rice)	stock/gravy/soup
	soy sauce	stir-fries
	tamari (wheat-free soy sauce)	stir-fries
	tempeh	stir-fry, roasted
	tofu (silken or firm)	soups, stews, stir-fry, grilled, smoothies, desserts
	yoghurt	yoghurt

A Week of Good Mood Meals

* = A Top Ten Good Mood Recipe (to be found in this handbook)
(MM) = part of the Mind Meal for mental health (*see Chapter 9*)

Seven Breakfast Ideas

1   Buckwheat porridge with almond nut butter and sugar-free blueberry jam
2   Puffed corn/cornflakes with fresh fruit, sunflower seeds and almond milk
3   Pumpernickel bread, toasted with tahini (sesame seed paste) and fruit spread*
4   Oat porridge with dried dates and oat milk
5   Toasted corn bread with cashew nut butter and sugar-free cherry jam
6   Wheat free muesli (make your own from oat, millet, buckwheat and rice flakes, dried fruit
     and nuts or buy ready-made) with an alternative milk of your choice
7   Millet porridge, dried apricots and rice milk*

Seven Lunch Ideas

1   Rice cakes, olives and hummus dip
2   Oil-rich fish with salad and corn chips/crisps/crackers
3   Rye crackers and vegetable/lentil pâté
4   Corn bread toasted with pesto sauce as spread
5   Grilled/Broiled sardines on corn/maize bread*
6   Baked beans (sugar-free brand) on wholegrain rye toast
7   Avocado salad and toasted seeds (MM)

Seven Dinner Ideas

1   Wheat-free pasta and oil-rich fish (MM)
2   Chicken stir-fry with buckwheat noodles
3   Buckwheat and lentils*
4   Jacket potato, fresh tuna and sweetcorn
5   Creamy turkey or chicken rainbow salad*
6   Basmati rice with flaked fish and peas*
7   Three bean vegetable casserole

Seven Dessert/Snack Ideas

1   Rice flake delight*
2   Fruit flapjack*
3   Stewed fruit on oatcakes (MM)
4   Sweet potato cakes*
5   Carob smoothie*
6   Fruit salad with nuts and seeds
7   Baked banana and nut butter

10 Good Mood Take-out Snacks

What do you do if you are out and about (without your own provisions), need something quick to eat and want a healthy alternative that also avoids your problem foods? Here are 10 'emergency' take-out snacks and drinks that are often available, and which shouldn't contain the common culprit foods.

1   Baked potato (no butter)
2   Chips/French fries (thick chips made from real potatoes are healthier)
3   Decaff coffee (will contain some caffeine)
4   Flapjack (check that it is wheat-free)
5   Fruit
6   Herbal tea
7   Plain potato crisps (plain crisps avoid problem additives)
8   Nuts/trail mix (combination of dried fruit, nuts and seeds)
9   Popcorn (plain or choose variety without butter)
10   Vegetable rice (e.g. from an oriental restaurant)

Good Mood Food First Aid Kit

If you're serious about changing what you eat, it is a good idea to carry some supplies around with you. Portable provisions help to avoid blood sugar lows that can throw your good mood (and good food intentions) off balance. Personal supplies can also 'bridge the gap' if, for example, you're out and away from food for longer than you anticipated.

- Dried apricots
- Dried figs
- Flapjack *(see recipe, page 128)*
- Fruit
- Herbal tea bags
- Nuts (try walnuts, almonds, Brazil nuts)
- Oat cakes (eat with dried fruit for an instant DIY 'flapjack' taste)
- Plain corn or potato chips/crisps
- Popcorn (try making your own and sprinkling with gomasio – sea salt and sesame seeds)
- Rice cakes
- Seeds (try plain or toasted sunflower or pumpkin seeds)
- Trail mix (your own delicious combination of dried fruit, nuts and seeds)

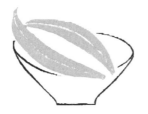

11

Feeling Good with Food

This chapter looks at some factors apart from food that can affect the state of the mind. It is important that the power of the mind and its expectations about the effects of food should not be overlooked during your exploration into food and mood.

Mind Power

We need to place more value on how we feel inside, despite what we may have been told.

The positive power of expectation is known in the medical world as the 'placebo effect'. It is demonstrated through the use of 'dummy pills' which are known as 'placebo' medication. Even though placebo pills have no active ingredients, they are sometimes found to be an extremely effective form of medicine. In experiments to test the effectiveness of new drugs, for example, dummy pills (used as a comparison for 'real' pills) can sometimes provide genuine health benefits for patients as good as the 'real' medication. Volunteer patients who, expecting a real treatment and unaware that they have been 'tricked', still report benefits from taking the 'pretend' medicine.

If someone tells us something is going to affect the way we feel (or the opposite – that it won't affect us), it seems that we are likely to believe them, regardless of our inner experience of the substance. It appears that we need to respect the power of our minds. We also need to place more value on how we feel inside, despite what we may have been told. Experiments have shown, for example, that the effects on the mind of alcohol and amphetamines can be altered according to what is expected. In one experiment, volunteers became drunk on alcohol-free beer because they had been told the drink contained alcohol.

In another experiment, a group of volunteers took an amphetamine (speed) but were told they'd been given a dummy pill. Instead of enjoying the increased arousal (the experience normally expected), they felt only anxiety. Because the volunteers believed there would be no effect from the (real) pill they'd been given, the usual experience of taking the amphetamine had been changed. Our expectations seem able to alter our experience.

Scientific Research

To dismiss the food–mood connection could be potentially harmful.

So great is the power of the mind that, before any new medical treatment is considered to be worthwhile, it has to prove itself as being even more potent than this power of suggestion. Rigorous scientific testing of foods to find their effects on the mind needs to bypass the experimenters' and volunteers' expectations in some way. Hiding foods in capsules or, in a hospital setting, feeding it directly into the stomach to avoid the taste buds in the mouth, are two possible methods for this type of scientific inquiry into food and mood. But these methods are not without problems, and the difficulties of conducting food–mood experiments may be what is currently deterring scientists from carrying out the much-needed research.

Meanwhile, to continue to dismiss the food–mood connection could be potentially harmful. Bliss from such ignorance is one thing, but unexplained anxiety or depression (for example) is quite another. Fortunately, many individuals are able to find out for themselves how what they eat affects how they feel, and need not wait for scientific evidence to confirm the power of food on the mind. By becoming aware of the effect food has upon your moods – even without making any long-term changes to what you eat – you gain greater self-knowledge which can give you more choice and more control over how you feel.

Food Choices

Emotional and social factors as well as practical and financial issues can play a part every time we decide what to eat and drink.

There are many influences behind the choices we make about food and eating. Many people feel they have a strong connection with food – a relationship that is a source of pleasure for some yet more painful for others. Emotional and social factors as well as practical and financial issues can play a part every time we decide what to eat and drink. This section takes a look at some of the emotional and social ingredients that are 'in the mix' when we make decisions about food. The exercise below can help with the exploration of your social and emotional relationship with food.

Food and Mood and You

The relationship between food and mood works both ways and there are many factors influencing what we choose to eat and drink. It is helpful to be aware of as many of these as possible so that we can take greater control of them and start to make more informed choices about our diet. When it comes to your relationship with food, how well do you know yourself? Here are some questions that Food & Mood Project participants have considered, which you may also like to think about.

1   What is your favourite food? Why do you think you like it so much?
2   Name any food(s) you like so much you can find yourself craving. When are you most likely to want these foods?
3   Which foods do you dislike? Why do you think you dislike them so much?
4   What would be your favourite meal? Describe it in detail, including the setting and who (if anyone) is there with you.
5   Complete this sentence for as many examples of feelings and food as you can: 'When I feel _____ I like to eat/drink _____'
6   Complete this sentence for as many examples of food and feelings as you can: 'When I eat/drink _____ I feel _____'
7   What routines, rituals or rules do you have around food (e.g. 'I always start the day with a cup of tea', 'I always have a glass of wine after an argument', 'You should always eat a cooked meal every day')? Which of these do you find helpful? Which may not be as beneficial for you?
8   Think of words or phrases that describe what food means (or meant) to you a) as a child, b) as an adult, c) as a food provider or parent (e.g. as a child food meant: 'arguments', 'being spoilt', 'no choice'; as an adult food means: 'more control', 'worries about health', 'free to choose'; as a parent/provider of food: 'responsibility', 'pleasure of giving', 'concern about cost of food'). Are you aware of any connections between your feelings about food now and when you were a child?
9   In your experience, how has food been used to show emotions such as love, as a comfort,

to show disapproval, as a reward/incentive, as a bribe, instead of giving attention, to relieve boredom, to upset someone? ('Mum worked when I was little and I missed her when I got home from school. But she'd always come home later with a cake or sweets for us. It felt like she was trying to make up for the fact she wasn't there by giving us food. I still have mixed feelings about the particular cakes and sweets that I associate with that time.' 'Stuffing down the feelings by comfort eating'. 'Thinking that the way to a man's heart is "through his stomach" and cooking him an impressive dinner'.)

There are no 'right' or 'wrong' answers to these questions. Instead it is the process of thinking about food, and perhaps writing down these thoughts and feelings, that helps you to become more aware of the complexity of your relationship with food. You may find it helpful to do this exercise with a friend and then share your answers with each other. You could also repeat this exercise some weeks or months later and notice how your answers have changed.

Blocks to Better Eating

Many people already have some idea of how they could improve their diets but find it difficult to change. When asked what prevents them from making the changes they wanted, the reasons given by Food and Mood Project participants ranged from emotional

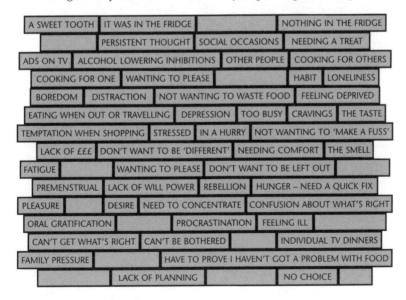

Fig 28 – Blocks to better eating brick wall

and social considerations to practical and financial constraints. Some of these 'blocks to better eating' are shown here, appropriately in the form of a brick wall. How many of these can you identify with? Are there any more that you could add?

Food Problems? Some Solutions

Solutions to the problems of changing what we eat were also discussed by Food and Mood Project participants. A selection of their suggestions is offered here, represented optimistically as leaves growing on a tree. This image can remind us that solutions to problems tend to emerge naturally, in their own time and season. Maybe you can add some 'leaves' of your own?

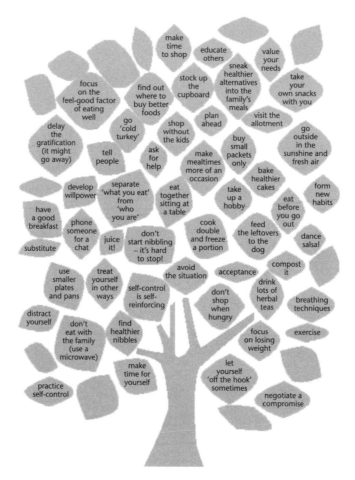

Fig 29 – Solutions 'tree'

Eating Intuitively

The increase in self-awareness that is needed for an effective exploration into the relationship between food and mood may lead you towards the idea of eating intuitively. Intuitive eating does not discount information we have heard or learned from other people but links it with a source of wisdom from deep within ourselves. Nevertheless, intuitive decisions about food can appear to fly in the face of what we may have been assuming is right for us to eat. Eating intuitively is a skill that, for many, takes time to develop. It involves learning to distinguish between impulses, hunger sensations and cravings that are the result of food sensitivities or an addictive-type relationship with food, and those that represent a genuine need for nutrients.

The senses of smell and taste, which are closely linked, form the guide to making intuitive choices between foods. What appeals to these senses is assumed to be beneficial for the body-mind. Intuitive decisions are helped by comparing the smell (and possibly the taste) of a range of alternative foods in an exercise which clarifies how attractive or not something is to these senses. In other words, you are able to judge more accurately what appeals to you when you can compare the smell (and/or taste) of two or more foods or drinks.

It is generally assumed (although this may not necessarily be the case) that intuitive choices are more accurate if the foods being sampled are in their raw, uncooked state. Thus, advocates of intuitive eating tend to recommend moving towards a predominantly raw food diet, primarily because of the higher nutrient content of raw foods. However, whether a raw food diet is always going to be desirable or more beneficial is debatable.

To take intuitive eating further, you can start by giving yourself time to pay attention to the smells and tastes of foods as you prepare a meal.

The skills of intuitive eating will be developed through adopting the approaches used in this handbook. To take intuitive eating further you can start by giving yourself time to pay attention to the smells and tastes of foods as you prepare a meal. Even choosing a drink provides an opportunity to exercise intuitive eating skills. Simply give yourself two or three tea bags or jars to smell or sample and notice how you feel when you experience them. Be aware of physical sensations as well as an emotional response. You are likely to find that what appeals one day will change, as the needs of your body alter over time. Intuitive eating is a process of paying attention to how your body-mind feels about food.

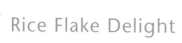

Rice Flake Delight

Type:	Dessert
Equipment:	medium pan, hob, liquidizer/blender (for almond milk)
Preparation time:	1 min
Cooking time:	8 mins

Finding a dessert that is as convenient as a pot of yoghurt when on a dairy- and soya-free diet can be challenging. Rice Flake Delight could be the solution as it can be enjoyed warm or chilled. It is so versatile it can be used as a breakfast porridge or a late-night snack. This recipe uses dried figs but any dried or fresh fruit can be substituted to suit individual taste. Figs are good for maintaining a healthy gut-brain connection and are also a good source of good mood minerals magnesium, manganese and potassium. Almond milk can be purchased from health-foods stores but is easy to make at home (see instructions below). Some people like to soak whole almonds overnight to activate the enzymes present in the nut which can help with digestion. Blanched, chopped or ground almonds can also be used. This milk can keep in the fridge but is best made immediately prior to use. It does need a shake before pouring as it separates on standing. To make almond 'cream', simply use less water. Almond milk is not suitable for young children.

Ingredients (per person)

For almond milk:
300ml/½ pint/1 cup water
25g/1oz/¼ cup almonds

1–2 dried figs, preferably preservative-free
90g/3½oz/1 cup brown rice flakes
300ml/½ pint/1 cup almond milk/rice milk
1 tbsp pinenuts
1 tbsp linseeds

Method

1   To make almond milk, simply blend almonds with water. If preferred, strain to remove small nut pieces.
2   Snip dried figs with scissors to make pea-sized pieces.
3   Place all ingredients into pan and heat on a medium heat, stirring occasionally. Add more milk if it starts to stick and to get the preferred consistency.
4   When ready, transfer to individual bowls and enjoy. Alternatively, chill in fridge to eat cold later on.

Ready?

Underdone	Rice flakes still separate and swimming in milk.
Just right	Flakes have merged with milk to create creamy consistency.
Overdone	Mixture sticking to pan and starting to burn.
Trouble-shooting tips	Too much liquid: simmer until excess has evaporated.
	Too dry: add more milk.

The Importance of Breathing

Strange though it may seem at first, but eating, breathing and feeling are all intimately connected. Many symptoms such as anxiety, depression, irritability and fatigue may have more to do with the way you are breathing than what you are eating. You may have adopted an unconscious breathing pattern to counterbalance the negative effects of certain foods. This is because the way we breathe and what we eat can affect the delicate acid–alkali balance of the cells and tissues of the body. An excess of either acidity or alkalinity will cause us to feel under stress, so it is necessary to maintain a balance between the two extremes if we are to feel good. Chapter 3 lists foods that are either acid- or alkali-forming. Here we shall pay attention to how we are breathing.

How Are You Breathing?

Try this simple exercise to discover your natural way of breathing.

1   Find a place where you can sit comfortably and undisturbed for a few minutes.
2   Close your eyes and focus on how you are breathing.
3   Place one hand on your chest and the other on your abdomen (belly area).
4   Notice how each hand moves as you continue to breathe in and out in your usual way. Does your upper hand, resting on your chest, move more than the hand that is resting on your abdomen? Do they move about the same amount or does the lower hand that is resting on your belly move more?
5   Let your hands fall so that they rest in your lap and slowly open your eyes.

This exercise shows how you are breathing. If your upper hand moved more than the lower hand resting on your abdomen, you are probably a habitual 'chest-breather' rather than a habitual 'belly-breather'. This type of upper chest breathing is normally reserved for coping with stressful situations and is very effective for increasing the amount of oxygen that is needed at these times. Unfortunately, breathing this way in the long term tends to convince the body that it is under a constant state of stress. The excess oxygen and relative lack of carbon dioxide causes the blood to become over-alkaline and symptoms resembling food sensitivity and then chronic illnesses can develop.

You can begin to change from being a chest-breather to a belly-breather by using the simple exercise below.

Belly-breathing

Sit quietly and close your eyes, if it helps you to focus. Notice how you are breathing. Imagine that a few inches from your lips is a lighted candle. As you breathe out, purse your lips as if you were going to blow out the candle flame. Exhale slowly in such a way that (if it were really there) you would gently blow the candle flame so that it flickered but did not blow out. Inhale and repeat the imaginary candle-blowing-out-but-not-quite exhalation. Continue for a few more cycles of inhalation and exhalation and then return to your normal breathing pattern. Notice if you feel any different. This simple exercise has the effect of extending the out-breath which will benefit your body's acid–alkali balance and leave you feeling more calm and relaxed.

Tips for Stress-free Eating

- Your body will be able to digest the meal better and absorb (and then use) more of the nutrients from your food if you can avoid eating whilst feeling stressed. So try sitting down to eat, turning off the phone, putting on some relaxing music and taking time to enjoy your meal.
- Eat slowly and chew your food well – your stomach doesn't have teeth and needs all the help it can get to start the process of digestion.
- It is preferable to reduce the amount of water or other liquids consumed with a meal as these can dilute digestive juices.
- Finally, if you want a coffee after your meal, you could try a caffeine-free alternative available from health-food stores. Caffeine-containing drinks are best drunk one hour after a meal as they reduce absorption of essential good mood minerals from food.

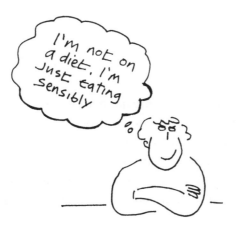

Wise Words

Principles of good nutrition:

- Give praise
- Eat that which is fresh
- Eat that which is in season
- Eat in measure

- Taste what you eat
- Enjoy what you eat
- Be thankful

Based on the principles of the Indian system of Ayurveda (the knowledge of life).

Self-help Groups

If you don't want to make changes to your diet alone and can't access professional help, a self-help group may be the answer. For people interested in exploring the relationship between what they eat and how they feel, self-help groups can provide much support and motivation. By including a good mood food-tasting session as part of your meetings you can encourage people to come along. This shared food-tasting experience also reduces the financial risk for individuals who may buy new food to try, only to find that they don't like it and then feel they've wasted their money. With a range of goodies on offer and several people to take part in the tasting, it is likely that there will be something for everyone to take home with them. If this idea appeals, you could start by contacting the organizations listed in the Resources section to see if there are any such groups available for you to join. If there aren't, you may be able to get help in starting one.

Eating Disorders

Compulsive eating, bulimia and anorexia nervosa are forms of eating distress. Compulsive eaters may feel they have no control over the amount they eat and can develop health problems associated with obesity. People suffering with anorexia often have a very distorted perception of their appearance and will continue to want to lose weight and deny themselves food even though they are already considerably underweight. Those suffering from bulimia tend to alternate between binge-eating and the need to get rid of food they have eaten, sometimes by vomiting, using laxatives, excessive fasting or exercise. Although these eating disorders can have associated nutritional deficiencies and are illnesses that can be made worse by having food sensitivities, they also have a powerful psychological component. They are serious and potentially dangerous conditions which need expert help, preferably from someone who is aware of the nutritional as well as the psychological factors involved.

Final Thoughts

This handbook has explored, in some detail, how you can investigate the food–mood connection. Yet the underlying ideas and assumptions are quite simple and, in conclusion, they are summarized below:

Guiding Principles

- The food and mood relationship works both ways: how you feel influences what you eat and drink, and what you eat and drink can affect how you feel.
- Precisely how food affects mood will vary from person to person.
- For any individual, the effects of food on mood are likely to change over time.
- A process of self-reflection in combination with careful, step-by-step changes to what you eat and drink should reveal how foods can affect your moods.
- Changing what you eat (and drink) will mean eating more of some foods and less of others.
- The food–mood exploration will be easier if you can enjoy the process of experimentation and change.

This handbook has encouraged you to consider how food can feed the mind as well as the body. It recommends that diet and nutrition are recognized as an essential part of caring for emotional and mental health. The mind, body and the food we eat are seen as closely connected, and may not be as separate as once believed. It is hoped that you can eat well and enjoy what you eat because you will now know from your own experience how food can influence your mood.

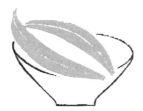

Resources

The following are sources of further information or assistance. The details were correct at the time of publication but may have changed since.

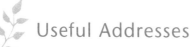

Useful Addresses

The Food & Mood Project
PO Box 2737, Lewes, BN7 2GN
Produces a quarterly newsletter and runs Food & Mood talks, courses and workshops. An on-line support group and private consultations are also available. Please send an s.a.e. for information or visit www.foodandmood.org

Practitioners (UK)

If you would like help in exploring the food and mood connection, it is recommended you contact a registered nutritional therapist. In the UK you will need to contact the British Association of Nutritional Therapists (BANT) who hold a nationwide list of registered nutritional therapists. Please contact BANT, 27 Old Gloucester Street, London, WC1N 3XX. Tel/Fax: 0870 606 1284.

The following BANT members have confirmed they are experienced in working with clients whose symptoms include emotional difficulties such as anxiety or depression and/or with clients who have a diagnosed mental illness. These practitioners may be contacted directly.

Although face-to-face consultations are preferable, many also offer a 'postal' or telephone consultation service.

Barrie Anson
Rowan House, 2 Malherbie Court, Knowle St Giles, Chard, Somerset TA20 4AZ
Tel: 01460 63238, e-mail: barrie.anson@virgin.net
Experience in treating: anxiety, depression, emotional difficulties, fears, phobias.

Linda Barr
The Nutrition & Health Co. Ltd., 3 Knockhundred Row, Midhurst,
West Sussex GU29 9DQ
Tel: 01730 814943, e-mail: LindaSBarr@aol.com, www.nutrition-healthco.com
Clinic also in Christchurch.

Christine Blakey
Pathways, 17a Blacket Place, Edinburgh EH9 1RJ
Tel: 0131 662 4088, e-mail: PathwaysHC@aol.com

June Butlin
Centre for Nutritional Excellence, 34 Magnolia Rise, West Ashton Road,
Trowbridge, Wiltshire BA14 7SJ
Tel: 01225 754924, e-mail: nutexcelezoom.co.uk, www.nutritional-excellence.com
Experience in treating: ADHD, Alzheimer's, anxiety, depression, eating disorders,
Parkinson's, schizophrenia, children.

Mary Cannon
Watling Street Therapy Centre, 24 Watling Street, Canterbury, Kent CT1 2UB
Tel: 01227 452202/830596, e-mail: mary.cannon@virgin.net
Clinics also at Margate and Deal.

Pam England
6 St Margaret's Road, Oxford OX2 6RU
Tel: 01865 510054, e-mail: pam-e@nildram.co.uk
Experience in treating: anxiety, bipolar disorder, depression, eating disorders.

Michael Franklin
137 Magdalen Road, Oxford OX4 1RJ
Tel: 01865 248403, e-mail: mfranklin@allergysolutions.fsnet.co.uk
Experience in treating: anxiety, chronic fatigue syndrome (ME), depression, mood
swings, eating disorders, PMS.

John Googe
Nutrition Advice Ltd, 32 Trent Court, New Wanstead, London E11 2TF
Tel: 020 8989 1812

Julie Green

The Health Team, Crown Treatment Centre, 2 Crown Lane, Littleport, Ely, Cambridgeshire CB6 1PP

Tel: 08707 898909

Mary Halliday

Kentrigg, St John's Park, Menston, Ilkley, West Yorkshire LS29 6ES

Tel: 01943 874769

Jenny Hargreaves

Lasata, Laurel's Avenue, Bangor on Dee, Wrexham LL13 0BB

Tel: 01978 7801216

Clinics also at Shewsbury and Oswestry.

Joy Healey

34 Kynaston Wood, Harrow HA3 6UA

Tel: 020 8954 9995

Pamela Jones

Springwood, Chivery, Nr Tring, Herts HP23 6LD

Tel: 01296 696333, e-mail: nutritionist@compuserve.com

Experience in treating: eating disorders.

Heather Lyons

43 Bow Fell, Rugby, Warwickshire CV21 1JF

Tel: 01778 552288

Lorraine Perretta

Nutrition Consulting Services, 60 Kenyon Street, London SW6 6LB

Tel: 020 7381 0688, e-mail: NEWTRIENT@AOL.COM

Experience in treating: depression, manic depression, OCD, schizophrenia.

Deidre Ramsey

Pippin's Couch, 121 City Road, Haverfordwest, Pembrokeshire SA61 2RR

Tel: 01437 768730, e-mail: 01437 768730

Experience in treating: autism, depression, eating disorders, OCD, PMS, schizophrenia.

Pat Reeves
Nutritional Cancer Therapy Trust, Oakfield Cottage, Bromley Lane, Kingswinford,
West Midlands DY6 8JP
Tel: 01384 270270, e-mail: pat@reeves-online.fsnet.co.uk, www.reeves-online.fesnet.co.uk
Experience in treating: experiential knowledge of emotional healing for all
mind/body/spirit disorders.

Catherine Smith
Brynawel, Trefonen, Oswestry, Shropshire SY10 9DQ
Tel: 01691 671514

Mary Strugar
The Nutrition Centre, 97 Harberton Road, London N19 3JT
Tel: 0207 272 2920, e-mail: MRStrugar@aol.com

Mary Stuart
4 Whiston House, Goldsmith's Row, London E2 8SJ
Tel: 020 7739 8497

John Tunnicliff
London Nutrition Clinic, 6 Ashbridge Road, London E11 1NH
Tel: 020 8518 8442, www.nutriserve.com
Experience in treating: chronic fatigue syndrome (ME), depression, menopause, PMS,
schizophrenia.

Martina Watts
The Crescent Clinic of Complementary Medicine, 37 Vernon Terrace, Brighton,
East Sussex BN1 3JH
Tel: 01273 202221, e-mail: martina_watts@compuserve.com
Experience in treating: adults and children with behavioural, digestive and immune
problems.

Erica White
Nutritionhelp, 22 Leigh Hall Road, Leigh-on-Sea, Essex SS9 1RN
Tel: 01702 472085, e-mail: reception@nutritionhelp.com, www.nutritionhelp.com
Experience in treating: emotional disorders arising from yeast overgrowth (candidiasis),
chronic fatigue syndrome (ME), eating disorders.

Veronica Wolseley

Brecon Complementary Medicine Centre, Ty Henry Vaughan, Bridge Street, Brecon, Powys LD3 8AH

Tel: 01497 821301

Clinics also at Leominster and Hay-on-Wye. Talks & workshops also offered. Experience in treating: anxiety, bi-polar disorder, chronic fatigue syndrome (ME), depression, eating disorders, schizophrenia.

Practitioners (USA)

The following organizations can provide lists of practitioners:

American Academy of Environmenal Medicine

6333 Long, Suite 200–14, Shawnee K 66216.

4510 W. 89th Street, Prairie Village, Kansas 66207.

Tel: (913) 341 3625/248 0067

American Association of Naturopathic Physicians

PO Box 20386, Seattle, Washington 98102

Tel: (206) 323 7610, Fax: (206) 323 7612

American Holistic Medical Association

4101 Lake Boone Trail, Suite 201, Raleigh, NC 27607

Tel: (206) 323 7610

American Naturopathic Medical Association

PO Box 96273, Las Vegas, Nev 89193

Tel: (702) 897 7053

American Preventive Medical Association

PO Box 2111, Tacoma, WA 98401

Tel: (206) 926 0551, Fax: (303) 417 9378

Practitioners (Australia)

Australasian College of Nutritional & Environmental Medicine

13 Hilton Street, Beaumaris, Victoria 3193

Tel: 9589 6088

Can provide list of practitioners.

Australian Natural Therapists Association
PO Box 308, Melrose Park, South Australia 5039
Tel: 8297 9533/8371 3222, Fax: 8297 0003
Can provide list of practitioners.

Australian Naturopathic Practitioners and Chiropractors Association
1st Floor, 609 Camberwell Road, Camberwell, VIC 3124
Tel: 9889 0448

Australian Society for Environmental Medicine
2–11 Howell Close, Doncaster East, 3109 Victoria
Tel: 9842 1886
Can provide list of practitioners.

Naturopathic Physicians Association of Australia Inc.
2 Beaumont Road, Canterbury, VIC 3126
Tel: 9589 6088

Organizations

Action Against Allergy
PO Box 278, Twickenham, Middlesex TW1 4QQ
Tel: 020 8892 2711

Action for ME
PO Box 1302, Wells BA5 1YE
Tel: 01749 670799

Allergy Induced Autism (AIA)
3 Palmera Avenue, Calcot, Reading, Berks RG3 7DZ
Tel: 0121 444 6450, www.demon.co.uk/charities/AIA/aia.htm
Provides information on the link between food allergies and autism.

Allergy Research Foundation
PO Box 18, Aylesbury, Buckinghamshire HP22 4XJ
Tel: 01296 655818, Fax: 020 7380 9351

Autism Research Unit
School of Health Sciences, University of Sunderland, Sunderland SR2 7EE
Tel: 0191 510 8922, Fax: 0191 567 0420, e-mail: aru@sunderland.ac.uk,
www.osiris.sunderland.ac.uk/autism

Berrydales
Berrydale House, 5 Lawn Road, London NW3 2XS
Tel: 020 7722 2866, Fax: 020 7722 7685, www.inside-story.com

British Allergy Foundation
Deepdene House, 30 Bellegrove Road, Welling, Kent DA16 3YP
Tel: 020 8303 8525

British Society for Allergy, Environmental and Nutritional Medicine (BSAENM)
PO Box 28, Totton, Southampton SO40 2ZA
Tel: 01703 812124, Fax: 01703 813912

Eating Disorders Association (EDA)
Sackville Place, 44 Magdalene Street, Norwich NR3 1IU
01603 619 090 (admin), 01603 621 414 (helpline)
Information and support for people with eating disorders.

The Hyperactive Children's Support Group (HACSG)
71 Wyke Lane, Chichester, East Sussex PO19 2LD
Tel: 01903 725182, www.hacsg.org
Information on the role of diet and nutrition in hyperactivity and ADHD.

ME Association
4 Corringham Road, Stanford-le-Hope, Essex SS17 OHA
Tel: 01375 642 466

Mental Health Foundation
20/21 Cornwall Terrace, London NW1 4QL
Tel: 020 7535 7400, Fax: 020 7535 7474

Mental Health Foundation (Scotland)
24 George Square, Glasgow G2 1EG
Tel: 0141 572 0125, Fax: 0141 572 0246, www.mhf.org.uk

Mind (National Association for Mental Health)
15–19 Broadway, London E15 4BQ
Tel: 020 8519 2122, www.mind.org.uk

Northern Ireland Association for Mental Health
Central Office, Beacon House, 80 University Street, Belfast BT7 1HE
Tel: 02890 328474

North West Mind
21 Ribblesdale Place, Preston PR1 3NA
Tel: 01772 821734

Northern Mind
Pinetree Centre, Durham Road, Birtley, Chester-le-Street, County Durham DH3 2TD
Tel: 0191 490 0109

South East Mind
1st Floor, Kemp House, 152–160 City Road, London EC1V 2NP
Tel: 0171 608 0881

South West Mind
Pembroke House, 7 Brunswick Square, Bristol BS2 8PE
Tel: 0117 925 0960

Trent & Yorkshire Mind
44 Howard Street, Sheffield S1 2LX
Tel: 0114 272 1742

West Midlands Mind
20–21 Cleveland Street, Wolverhampton WV1 3HT
Tel: 01902 424404

Mind Cymru
3rd Floor, Quebec House, Castlebridge, Cowbridge Road East, Cardiff CF11 9AB
Tel: 01222 395123

Schizophrenia Association of Great Britain
International Schizophrenia Association, Bryn Hyfrd, The Crescent, Bangor,
Gwynnedd LL57 2SAG
Tel: 01248 354048, e-mail: sagb@btinternet.com, www.btinternet.com/~sagb

Sustain – the alliance for better food and farming
94 White Lion Street, London N1 9PF
Tel: 020 7837 1228, Fax: 020 7837 1141, www.sustainweb.org

York Nutritional Laboratory
Murton Way, Osbaldwick, York YO19 5US
Tel: 01904 690640, www.allergy-testing.com
Provides an allergy-testing service by post.

Alternative Food Sources (UK)

The customer services department of food stores hold lists of products which are free from certain ingredients suitable for those on special diets.

Asda	0500 1000055	Safeway	01622 712899
Boots	0115 9506111	Somerfield	0117 935 9359
Co-op	0800 0686727	Tesco	0800 505555
Marks & Spencer	020 7268 1234	Waitrose	01344 824975
Sainsbury	0800 636262		

Against the Grain Ltd
Claridge House, 29 Barnes High Street, London SW13 9LW
Tel: 020 8876 6247

AllergyCare
1 Church Square, Taunton, Somerset TA1 1SA.
Tel: 01823 325023

Allergyfree Direct Ltd.
5 CentreMead, Osney Mead OX2 0ES
Tel: 01865 722003, Fax: 01865 244134, www.allergyfreedirect.co.uk

Barbara's Kitchen
PO Box 54, Pontyclun, South Wales CF72 8WD
Tel: 01443 229304, e-mail: enquiries@barbara'skitchen.co.uk, www.barbaraskitchen.co.uk

Blissful Buffalo (milk and meat)
Belland Farm, Tetcott, Holsworthy, Devon EX22 6RG
Tel: 01409 271406, www.Blissfulbuffalo.fsnet.co.uk

Buxton Foods Ltd.
12 Harley Street, London W1N 1AA
Tel: 020 7637 5505, Fax: 020 7436 0979, e-mail: sales@stamp-collection.co.uk, www.stamp-collection.co.uk

D & D Specialist Chocolates
261 Forest Road, Loughborough LE11 3HT
Tel: 01509 216400, Fax: 01509 233961

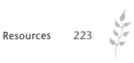

Delamere Direct (goat's milk)

Yew Tree Farm, Bexton Lane, Knutsford, Cheshire WA16 9BH

Tel: 01565 632422, e-mail: sales@delameredairy.co.uk, www.delameredairy.co.uk

Dietary Specialities Direct

Freepost NWW 2474A, Warrington WA5 5ZW

Tel: 07041 544044, Fax: 07041 544055, e-mail: info@nutritionpoint.ltd.uk, www.glutenfree-dsdirect.co.uk

Eskley Sheep Milk

Llanbaddon Farm, Michaelchurt, Eskley, Hereford HR2 0PR

Tel: 01981 510294, e-mail: info@sheepmilk.co.uk, www.sheepmilk.co.uk

Everfresh Natural Foods

Gatehouse Close, Aylesbury, Buckinghamshire HP19 3DE

Tel: 01296 425333

General Dietary Ltd.

PO Box 38, Kingston upon Thames, Surrey KT2 7YP

Tel: 020 8942 8274, Fax: 020 8942 8274

Goodness Direct

PO Box 6049, Daventry NN11 4UY

Tel: 01327 871655, Fax: 01327 310528, e-mail: info@goodnessdirect.co.uk, www.goodnessdirect.co.uk

Hambleden Herbs (organic herbs)

Court Farm, Milverton, Somerset TA4 1NF

Tel: 01823 401104, Fax: 01823 401001, e-mail: info@hambledenherbs.co.uk, www.hambledenherbs.co.uk

Lifestyle Healthcare Limited

Centenary Business Park, Henley-on-Thames, Oxfordshire RG9 1DS

Tel: 01491 411767, Fax: 01491 571704, www.glutenfree.co.uk

Motherhemp Foods Ltd.

71 Bushey Lodge, Firle, Nr Lewes, East Sussex BN8 6LS

Tel: 01323 811909, Fax: 0207 691 7475, e-mail: info@motherhemp.com, www.motherhemp.com

Organics Direct

1–7 Willow Street, London EC2A 4BH

Tel: 020 7729 2828, Fax: 020 7729 0534, www.organicsdirect.com

Pure Organics Ltd.

Stockport Farm, Stockport Road, Amesbury, Wilts SP4 7LN

Tel: 0800 783 7535, Fax: 01980 626264, e-mail: mail@pure.organics.org,
www.organics.org

Seabrook Potato Crisps Ltd. (unsalted plain crisps mail order)

Seabrook House, Allerton, Bradford, West Yorkshire BD15 7QU

Tel: 01274 546405, Fax: 01274 542235

Sillfield Farm Products (gluten-free sausages mail order)

Sillfield Farm, Endmoor, Kendal, Cumbria LA8 OHZ

Tel: 015395 67609, Fax: 015395 67483, e-mail: enquiries@sillfield.co.uk,
www.sillfield.co.uk

Simply Organic Food Company Ltd

New Covent Garden Market, London SW8 5YY

Tel: 0845 1000 444, e-mail: orders@simplyorganic.net, www.simplyorganic.net

Taste of the Wild (mail order special foods)

4 Waterside Drive, Purley-on-Thames, Reading, Berkshire RG8 8AQ

Tel/Fax: 01189 542263, www.tasteofthewild.co.uk

The Village Bakery

Melmerby, Penrith, Cumbria CA10 1HE

Tel: 01768 881515, Fax: 01768 881848, e-mail: info@village-bakery.com,
www.village-bakery.com

Nutritional Supplements

The following recommended supplement companies sell their products direct to the
public via mail order:

BioCare Ltd.

Lakeside, 180 Lifford Lane, Kings Norton, Birmingham B30 3NT

Tel: 0120 433 3727, Fax: 0121 433 8705

Higher Nature
Burwash Common, East Sussex TN19 7LX
Tel: 01435 883484

The Nutri Centre
7 Park Crescent, London W1N 3HE
Tel: 020 7436 5122, Fax: 020 7436 5171, www.nutricentre.com

Further Reading

Anthony, H., Birtwistle, S., Eaton, K., Maberly, J. (1997) *Environmental Medicine in Clinical Practice* BSAENM Publications, Southampton, UK.

Ashford, N.A., & Miller, C.S. (1998) Second edition *Chemical Exposures* Van Nostrand Reinhold, New York.

Barnes, B. & Colquhoun, I. (1998) *Hyperactive Children* Thorsons, London.

Batmanghelidji, F. (1992) *Your body's many cries for water* Redwood Books, UK.

Bradley, D. (1998) *Hyperventilation Syndrome* Kyle Cathie Limited, London.

Braly, J. (1992) *Dr Braly's Food Allergy & Nutrition Revolution* Keats Publishing Inc, USA.

Brostoff, J. & Gamlin, L. (1989) *The Complete Guide to Food Allergy and Intolerance* Bloomsbury, London.

BSAENM (1994) *Effective Allergy Practice* British Society for Allergy, Environmental & Nutritional Medicine, Southampton, UK.

BSAENM (1995) *Effective Nutritional Medicine* British Society for Allergy, Environmental & Nutritional Medicine, Southampton, UK.

Budd, M. (2000) *Is Your Thyroid Making You Ill?* Thorsons, London.

Chaitow, L. (1991) *Thorsons Guide To Amino Acids* Thorsons, London.

Chaitow, L. (1996) *Candida Albicans* Thorsons, London.

Colbin, A. (1986) *Food & Healing* Ballantine Books, New York.

Cox, P. & Brusseau, P. (1997) *Secret Ingredients* Bantam Books, London.

DesMaisons, K. (1998) *Potatoes Not Prozac* Simon & Schuster UK Ltd., London.

Elgin, D. (1993) Revised edition *Voluntary Simplicity* Quill, William Morrow & Co.

Erasmus, U. (1993) *Fats that Heal, Fats That Kill* Alive Books, Canada.

Fairburn, C. (1995) *Overcoming Binge Eating* The Guildford Press, New York.

Gottschall, E. (1994) *Breaking the Vicious Cycle* Kirkton Press Ltd., Canada.

Graedon, J. & Graedon, T. (1995) *Deadly Drug Interactions* St Martin's Griffin, New York.

Greenfield, S. (2000) *Brain Story* BBC Worldwide Ltd., London.

Hoffman, R. (1997) *Attention Deficit Disorder* Keats Publishing Inc.

Holford, P. (1997) *The Optimum Nutrition Bible* Piatkus, London.

Holford, P. (1998) *100% Health* Piatkus, London.

Kirschmann, G. (1996) Fourth Edition *Nutrition Almanac* McGraw-Hill, New York.

Joneja, J. (1998) Second Edition *Food Allergies & Intolerances* J.A. Hall Publications Ltd, Vancouver, Canada.

Langley, G. Second Edition (1995) *Vegan Nutrition* The Vegan Society, UK.

Lazarides, L. (1997) *The Nutritional Health Bible* Thorsons, London.

Ledwards, C. (1992) *Women, Food & Health* South Manchester Nutrition and Dietetic Service, UK. (This is a teaching pack.)

Leeds, A., Brand Miller, J., Foster-Powell, K., Colagiuri, S. (1996) *The GI Factor* Hodder & Stoughton, London.

Leggett, D. Third edition (1997) *Helping Ourselves – A Guide to Traditional Chinese Food Energetics* Meridian Press, Totnes, UK.

Logue, A.W. (1991) Second Edition *The Psychology of Eating and Drinking* W.H. Freeman & Co, New York.

Lombard, J. & Germano, C. (1997) *The Brain Wellness Plan* Kensington Books, London.

Maberly, J. & Anthony, H. (1989) *Allergy : a practical guide to coping* The Crowood Press, Wiltshire, UK.

Mackarness, R. (1976) *Not All In The Mind* Pan Books Ltd., London.

Miller, S. & Knowler, K. (2000) *Feel Good Food* The Women's Press Ltd, London.

Mind (2000) *The Mind Guide to Food and Mood* Mind, London.

Murray, M. (1993) *The Healing Power of Foods* Prima Publishing, USA.

Murray, M.T. & Pizzorno, J.E. (1990) *Encyclopaedia of Natural Medicine* Little, Brown & Company (UK), London.

Orbach, S. (1993) Second Edition *Hunger Strike* Penguin Books, London.

Pert, C. (1997) *Molecules of Emotion* Simon & Schuster UK Ltd., London.

Pfeiffer, C. & Holford, P. (1996) *Mental Health & Illness – the nutrition connection* ION Press, London. A clear and thorough explanation of this important subject.

Philpott, W. & Kalita, D. (1980) *Brain Allergies: The Psycho Nutrient Conection* Keats Publishing Inc., USA.

Reader's Digest (1999) *Fighting Allergies* Reader's Digest, London.

Schaeffer, S. (1987) *Instinctive Nutrition* Celestial Arts, California.

Schauss, A. (1997) *Anorexia & Bulimia* Keats Publishing Inc., USA.

Schmidt, M. (1997) *Smart Fats* Frog Ltd, USA.

Sellar, W. (1992) *The Directory of Essential Oils* The CW Daniel Co Ltd., UK.

Seyle, H. (1976) *The Stress of Life* (Revised Edition), McGraw-Hill.

Werbach, M. (1987) *Nutritional Influences on Illness* Keats Publishing Inc., USA.

Cookbooks

Berriedale-Johnson, M. (1999) *The Allergyfree Cookbook* Thorsons, London.
Carter, P. 4th edition (1998) *An Allergy Cookbook* Ian Henry Publications Ltd,
    Essex/Players Press Inc, California.
Carter, J.& Edwards, A. (1997) *The Rotation Diet Cookbook* Element Books Ltd, London.
Cousins, B. (2000) *Cooking Without* Thorsons, London.
Lazarides, L. (2000) *The Gourmet Nutritional Therapy Cookbook* Waterfall 2000, London.

The following publishers produce newsletters and booklets for those on special diets:

Barbara's Kitchen, PO Box 54, Pontyclun, South Wales CF72 8WD, Tel: 01443 229304,
    www.barbara'skitchen.co.uk
Berrydales Publishers, 5 Lawn Road, London NW3 2XS, Tel: 020 7722 2866,
    Fax: 020 7722 7685, e-mail: berrydales@compuserve.com, www.inside-story.com
Merton Books, PO Box 279, Twickenham, Middlesex TW1 4XQ, Tel: 020 8892 4949,
    Fax: 020 8892 4950, www.merton-books.co.uk

The Food and Mood Project

If you would like to take part in the on-going programme of research co-ordinated by
The Food and Mood Project, please write enclosing a large SAE to:

Research
The Food and Mood Project
PO Box 2737
Lewes
East Sussex
BN7 2GN

You may also like to visit our website at: www.foodandmood.org

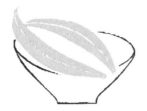

Index